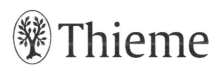

Color Atlas of Otology

Diagnosis and Management

Anirban Ghosh, MS-ENT
Chief Consultant
Hope Nursing Home
Raniganj, West Bengal, India

Thieme
Delhi • Stuttgart • New York • Rio de Janeiro

Publishing Director: Ritu Sharma
Development Editor: Dr. Ambika Kapoor
Director- Editorial Services: Rachna Sinha
Project Managers: Snehil Sharma
Vice President, Sales and Marketing: Arun Kumar Majji
Managing Director & CEO: Ajit Kohli

Thieme Medical and Scientific Publishers Private Limited.
A - 12, Second Floor, Sector - 2, Noida - 201 301, Uttar Pradesh, India, +911204556600
Email: customerservice@thieme.in
www.thieme.in

Cover design: Thieme Publishing Group
Typesetting by RECTO Graphics, India

Printed in India by Nutech Print Services

5 4 3 2 1

ISBN 978-93-90553-76-1
Also available as e-book:
eISBN 978-93-90553-77-8

Important note: Medicine is an ever-changing science undergoing continual development. Research and clinical experience are continually expanding our knowledge, in particular, our knowledge of proper treatment and drug therapy. Insofar as this book mentions any dosage or application, readers may rest assured that the authors, editors, and publishers have made every effort to ensure that such references are in accordance with **the state of knowledge at the time of production of the book.**

Nevertheless, this does not involve, imply, or express any guarantee or responsibility on the part of the publishers in respect to any dosage instructions and forms of applications stated in the book. **Every user is requested to examine carefully** the manufacturers' leaflets accompanying each drug and to check, if necessary, in consultation with a physician or specialist, whether the dosage schedules mentioned therein or the contraindications stated by the manufacturers differ from the statements made in the present book. Such examination is particularly important with drugs that are either rarely used or have been newly released in the market. Every dosage schedule or every form of application used is entirely at the user's own risk and responsibility. The authors and publishers request every user to report to the publishers any discrepancies or inaccuracies noticed. If errors in this work are found after publication, errata will be posted at www.thieme.com on the product description page.

Some of the product names, patents, and registered designs referred to in this book are in fact registered trademarks or proprietary names even though specific reference to this fact is not always made in the text. Therefore, the appearance of a name without designation as proprietary is not to be construed as a representation by the publisher that it is in the public domain.

My wife, Dr. Amrita, my pillar of strength, and my best friend
My kids Ahana and Abhirup, my bundle of joy
My parents, my source of inspiration

Anirban Ghosh

Contents

Foreword

It gives me great pleasure to write this foreword for *Color Atlas of Otology: Diagnosis and Management* by Dr. Anirban Ghosh.

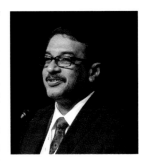

This atlas is a compendium of clinical photographs of the various diseases of the ear, painfully and meticulously collected over many years. It is scientifically accurate and exhaustive. Each photograph is also accompanied by a clear legend with detailed explanations about the condition, and notes on relevant management.

Common surgical procedures in otological practice are also outlined in the book with excellent photographs to illustrate each surgical step. This atlas is a labour of love and this is reflected in each and every chapter.

I have no doubt this book will immensely benefit both postgraduate and undergraduate students of otorhinolaryngology, as well as ENT and general practitioners.

I commend the author for this work of excellence. I am sure this atlas will find a place in every medical library.

I have no hesitation in commending this book in the highest terms.

Mohan Kameswaran, MBBS, DLO, MS, FRCS, FICS, DSc
Director
Madras ENT Research Foundation
Padmashri awardee
Chennai, Tamil Nadu, India

Foreword

It is a great pleasure for me to write this foreword for Dr. Anirban Ghosh. Learning is a lifelong process and Dr. Anirban is a strong believer in this statement. His desire to seek knowledge in the field of otology is unquenchable, and yes, that is how I know him! He has visited me more than eight times for the Temporal Bone workshop, making me ponder over his constant love for learning.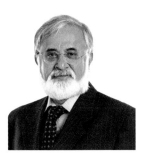

I appreciate his sincere efforts in achieving this commendable job of writing the monograph. This book is concise yet comprehensive in its illustrations for the junior trainees and colleagues, in diagnosing the common and rare otological diseases. The advent of the oto-endoscope is an adjuvant to the conventional approach of otological ailments. I must congratulate Dr. Anirban for such high-quality images that are self-explanatory and precise, and aid in better understanding.

The second part of the book describes common otological surgical procedures in a very systematic manner, highlighting the key tips and tricks. Moreover, his explanation of the subject in simple language makes it easier to comprehend the concepts, facts, and procedures. The attractive layout and organized presentation further assist in easy reading.

Although otology has made a great improvement in the country for the past few decades, I am certain that this monograph would help in its development at the international level. The chapter on imaging and postoperative complication management is worth reading for the budding trainees, young colleagues, and senior surgeons to be aware of the management in challenging situations.

I wish Dr. Anirban Ghosh all the luck for his future endeavors.

Dr. K. P. Morwani, MBBS, MS
Head, Department of ENT
Fortis Hiranandani Hospital
Mumbai, Maharashtra, India

Preface

Ear ailments are very common in all parts of the world, particularly in India. Patients present with earache, discharge, hearing loss, vertigo, and various other symptoms. Diagnosis of different otological diseases mostly depends on the physical examination of the tympanic membrane. Unfortunately, the narrow external auditory canal hinders the proper viewing of the tympanic membrane making the diagnosis even more difficult. The advent of the endoscope has revolutionized the field of otolaryngology. With better illumination and magnification, every nook and corner of the ear can be well visualized.

This book has been written in such a manner that healthcare professionals will benefit from the pictorial depiction of both normal anatomy of the ear, as well as its different pathologies. A chapter on otological surgeries has been included for residents and consultants, where detailed step-by-step illustrations of different surgical procedures have been given along with a discussion on every minute detail which will enable the surgeons to use it as a surgical road map for routine surgical procedures. The chapter on chronic otitis media with cholesteatoma requires a special mention. High-resolution computed tomography (HRCT) scan of temporal bone has improved our understanding of this disease pathology. HRCT has been very informative in cases of complicated chronic otitis media (squamous). My colleague Dr. Aniket Mondal has written a very informative chapter on this topic and I hope this will give the readers a new insight into the disease pathology. There is a chapter on postoperative results of different otological surgeries. One has to audit their surgical outcomes and document them to improve surgical results. This chapter will enlighten all otologists about postoperative complications and their management.

I hope this book will be a good companion to all consultants and postgraduate students dedicated towards improving the hearing of their patients.

Anirban Ghosh, MS-ENT

Acknowledgments

I express my sincere thanks to Dr. Aniket Mondal, MD, DNB, PDCC, Consultant Radiologist, Health World Hospital, Durgapur, West Bengal, India, for contributing a section on Radiology of the Ear for the book.

I thank my teacher Professor (Dr.) S. P. Bera for imbibing the essence of otology in my mind.

I also thank my teacher, friend, philosopher, and guide Professor (Dr.) Somnath Saha for constantly encouraging me.

Dr. K. P. Morwani, I am eternally indebted to you for engraving the finer aspects of otology in my mind. I was a silent observer of Dr. K. T. Patil's surgery and learned a lot from his surgical demonstrations.

I spent a few weeks with Professor (Dr.) Mohan Kameswaran at MERF, Chennai. I was enthralled by his dedication, knowledge, and humility.

I am grateful to my colleagues Dr. Sudipta Pal, Dr. Abhishek Srivastava, and Dr. Kanishka Chowdhury for constantly encouraging me.

I thank my friends Dr. Archana Singh and Dr. Mithun Choudhury for always standing beside me in most difficult times.

I thank Mr. Sandip Ruidas, Mr. Bholanath Mukherjee, and Mr. Niranjan Gope for helping me with documentation and scriptwriting.

I acknowledge the contribution of the staff at the operation theater of Hope Nursing Home, Mrs. Sikha, Jyotsna, Piyali, and Khusboo, for patiently assisting me and documenting images.

I sincerely thank my better half, Dr. Amrita, for patiently listening to the whole manuscript and providing inputs and corrections whenever required.

Lastly, I thank all my patients for their trust in me and for giving me the opportunity to serve them.

Anirban Ghosh, MS-ENT

Section A

Diseases of the Ear

1 Normal Auricle (External Ear)

Ear has been traditionally divided into external, middle, and inner ear. Different types of congenital, infective, traumatic, and neoplastic pathologies occur in the ear. This section consists of otoendoscopic pictures of different pathologies along with their description. Chapters have been divided into smaller sections depending on the pathology. All chapters have brilliant clinical images with short discussion that will help otologists and residents to have a pictorial idea about the disease.

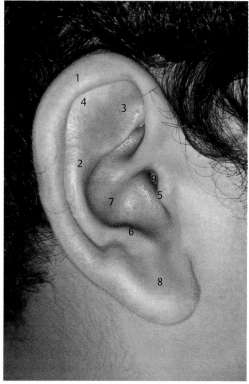

Fig. 1.1 Normal auricle. This is a normal appearing right ear. Landmarks are (1) helix, (2) antihelix, (3) triangular fossa, (4) scaphoid fossa, (5) tragus, (6) antitragus, (7) conchal bay, (8) lobule, and (9) external auditory meatus.

2 Diseases of the Auricle

2.1 Congenital Deformity

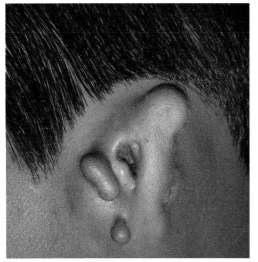

Fig. 2.1.1 Microtia. Congenital anomaly of external ear due to developmental abnormality of hillocks of His. This is Grade 3.

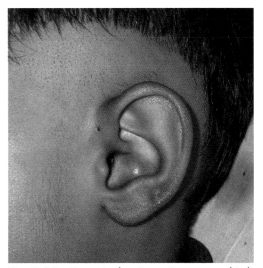

Fig. 2.1.2 Preauricular sinus. A common birth defect. Skin lined pit or hole in front of pinna, may be unilateral or bilateral. Swelling and pain with tenderness occur when it is infected. Antibiotic, pain killers are given for treatment of acute phase. Meticulous surgical excision after 4-6 weeks of medical treatment is the mainstay of treatment. Meticulous surgical excision is the treatment of choice. Here, it is in front of left ear.

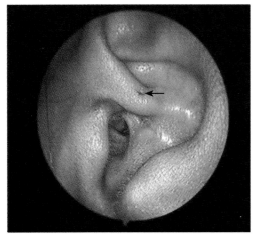

Fig. 2.1.3 Preauricular sinus at unusual site (left ear).

2.2. Inflammatory Diseases and Tumors of Auricle

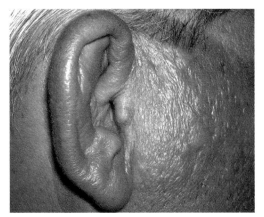

Fig. 2.2.1 Perichondritis of the right ear. Erythema, edema of the helical part of pinna, mostly due to trauma, infection. Must be treated with antibiotics.

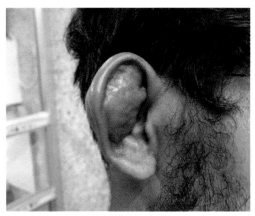

Fig. 2.2.2 Perichondrial abscess. Right-sided huge perichondrial abscess due to trauma.

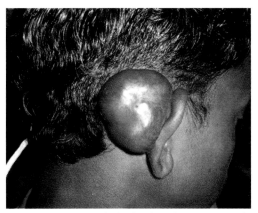

Fig. 2.2.3 Huge keloid of right ear, mostly due to trauma to the cartilage. It is treated with excision and intralesional steroid injection to reduce the chance of recurrence.

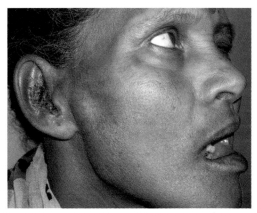

Fig. 2.2.4 Herpes zoster oticus right ear. Herpetic blisters noted in the right pinna with right-sided facial paralysis. It is called Ramsay-Hunt syndrome. It is treated with antiviral, steroid; prognosis of facial function improvement is 50 to 60%.

3 Diseases of External Auditory Canal

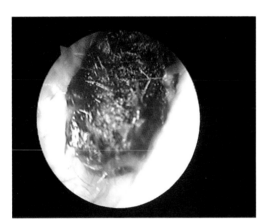

Fig. 3.1 Cerumen. It is produced by the secretion of ceruminous and sebaceous glands along with squamous debris. Normally we see either dry or wet type of cerumen. In both the cases, treatment is removal after proper ceruminolytic-drug local application.

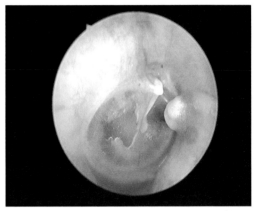

Fig. 3.2 Exostosis. It is a solitary bony overgrowth in the bony external canal. Here, it is in the anterior wall of the right ear. Usually, it is asymptomatic, but when it is large enough to block the tympanic membrane, then surgical removal becomes necessary.

3.1 Foreign Bodies

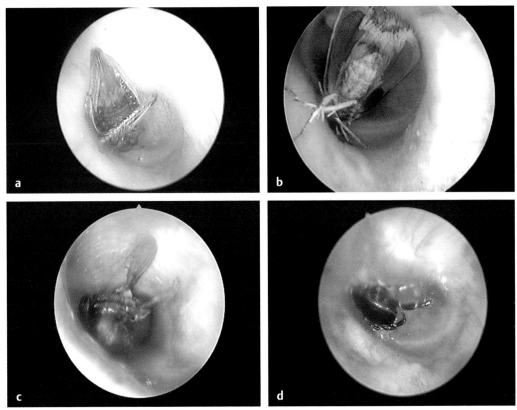

Figs. 3.1.1   (a–d) Different insects as foreign bodies.

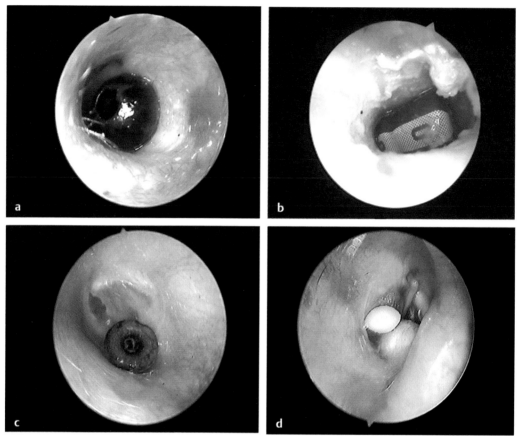

Figs. 3.1.2 (a–d) Different inanimate objects as foreign bodies.

3.2 Otomycosis

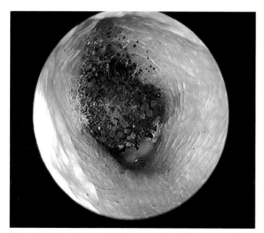

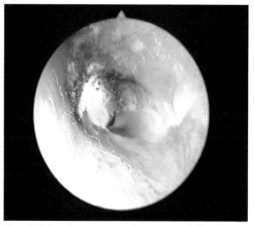

Fig. 3.2.1 Superficial mycotic infection of ear canal presented with discharge, inflammation, pain, and pruritus. *Aspergillus niger* appears as black-headed filamentous growth.

Fig. 3.2.2 Otomycosis due to *Candida albicans* seen as white, cheesy, and creamy deposits. Otomycosis is treated with topical antifungal followed by removal of it.

3.3 Other Inflammatory Diseases of External Auditory Canal

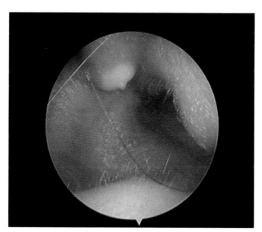

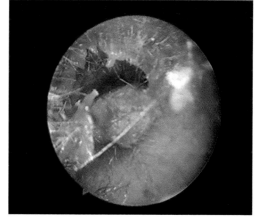

Fig. 3.3.1 Diffuse otitis externa (right ear). Diffuse otitis externa with furunculosis of right external auditory canal. It is due to Staphylococcal infection of hair follicle of external auditory canal (EAC).

Fig. 3.3.2 Seborrheic dermatitis. It is a skin disorder of hair follicle bearing external auditory canal (EAC) region. It is usually associated with seborrheic dermatitis of skin of other areas.

4 Normal Tympanic Membrane

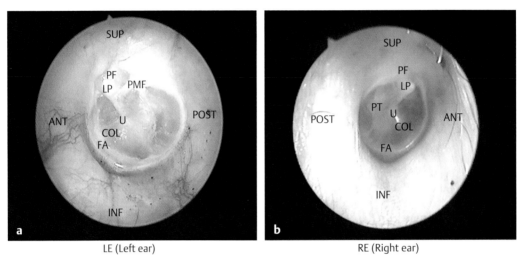

LE (Left ear)   RE (Right ear)

Fig. 4.1 (a, b) Normal tympanic membrane. ANT, anterior; COL, cone of light; FA, fibrous annulus; INF, inferior; LP, lateral process; PF, pars flaccida; PMF, posterior malleolar fold; POST, posterior; PT, pars tensa; SUP, superior; U, umbro.

5 Acute Inflammation of the Tympanic Membrane (Acute Otitis Media)

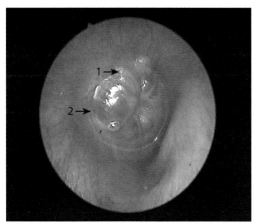

Fig. 5.1 Acute otitis media (AOM) of right ear: (1) showing congested handle of malleus; (2) suppuration with pus pushing pars tensa laterally.

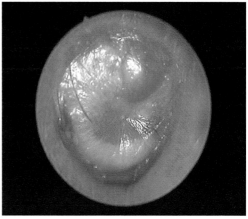

Fig. 5.2 Acute otitis media with congested vessels running toward umbo giving a cartwheel appearance with pus in the middle ear.

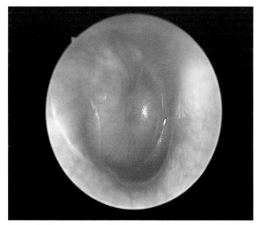

Fig. 5.3 Acute otitis media with cartwheel appearance and the middle ear is filled with pus.

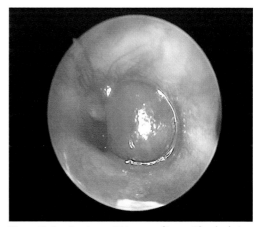

Fig. 5.4 Acute otitis media with bulging of tympanic membrane in posterosuperior quadrant.

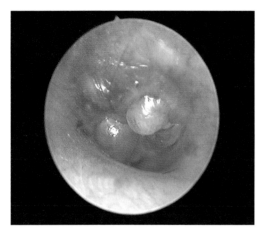

Fig. 5.5 Bullous myringitis: formation of multiple blisters.

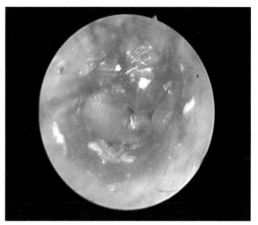

Fig. 5.6 Granular myringitis: localized chronic inflammation of outer surface of tympanic membrane with formation of granulation tissue which may lead to stenosis of deep external auditory canal.

6 Otitis Media with Effusion

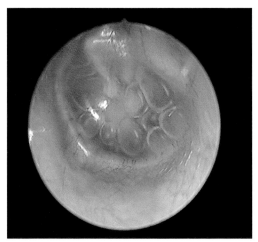

Fig. 6.1 Otitis media with effusion of left ear. There are multiple air bubbles inside the middle ear.

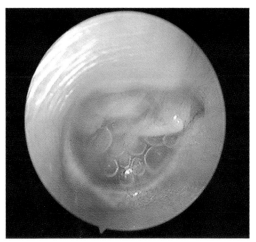

Fig. 6.2 Otitis media with effusion of right ear with air bubble.

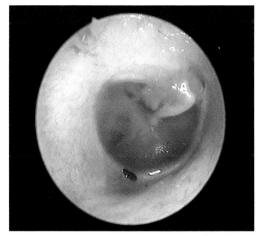

Fig. 6.3 Otitis media with effusion of right ear with absent cone of light and presence of fluid inside the middle ear.

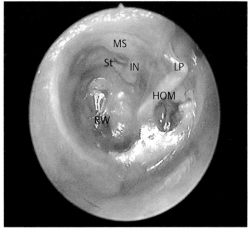

Fig. 6.4 Otitis media with effusion (OME) with retraction of right ear. Following OME, the air in the middle ear is sucked in, which leads to retraction of posterosuperior quadrant. Pars tensa touches incus, incudostapedial joint, stapedius, and round window. Myringosclerosis is noticed in the posterior superior quadrant. HOM, handle of malleus; IN, incus; LP, lateral process; MS, myringosclerosis; RW, round window; St, stapedius.

7 Retraction of the Tympanic Membrane

7.1 Retraction of Pars Tensa

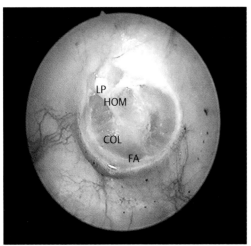

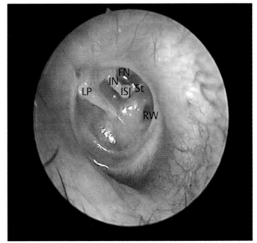

Fig. 7.1.1 Retraction of pars tensa is classified by Sade. Grade I of pars tensa retraction. Slight retraction of pars tensa, fibrous annulus (FA) becomes more prominent, cone of light (COL) is missing, lateral process (LP) of malleus is prominent due to unopposed medial pull of tensor tympani muscle leading to medialized handle of malleus (HOM).

Fig. 7.1.2 Grade II pars tensa retraction. Left ear showing Grade II retraction where pars tensa retracts and touches long process incus (IN). Here, we can see incudostapedial joint (ISJ), stapedius tendon (St), round window (RW), and part of horizontal facial nerve (FN). Lateral process of malleus (LP) is more prominent.

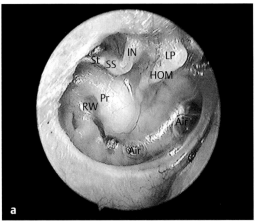
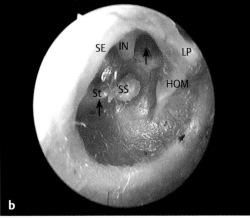

Fig. 7.1.3 **(a)** Grade III pars tensa retraction. Grade III retraction of pars tensa of right ear where pars tensa medializes more and adheres to promontory (Pr). It is called atelectatic tympanic membrane. Some air pockets (air) are still present in middle ear at anteroinferior and inferior quadrant. **(b)** Grade III retraction of pars tensa with incus necrosis and marked retraction pocket (*arrows*) between malleus-incus and posterior mesotympanum. HOM, handle of malleus; IN, incus; LP, lateral process; RW, round window; SS, stapes suprastructure; St, stapedius tendon.

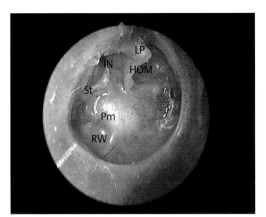
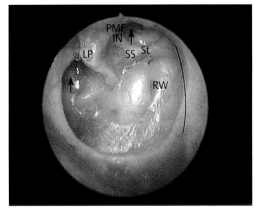

Fig. 7.1.4 Grade IV retraction of pars tensa. Further retraction of pars tensa leads to complete adhesion of tympanic membrane to promontory with no middle ear air. In this picture, there is Grade IV retraction of pars tensa (adhesive otitis media) with malleus retraction making lateral process (LP) prominent. Lenticular process incus (IN) is necrosed. Tympanic membrane is adhered to promontory (Pm)—with no middle ear air. HOM, handle of malleus; RW, round window; St, stapedius tendon.

Fig. 7.1.5 Grade IV pars tensa retraction. IN, incus; LP, lateral process; PMF, posterior malleolar fold; RW, round window; SS, stapes suprastructure; St, stapedius tendon.

7.2 Retraction of Pars Flaccida

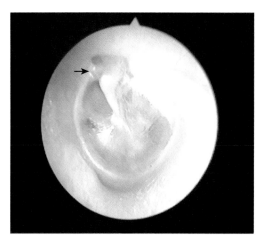

Fig. 7.2.1 Grade I retraction of pars flaccida, just a dimple (*arrow*) lateral to malleus with no bony erosion of scutum.

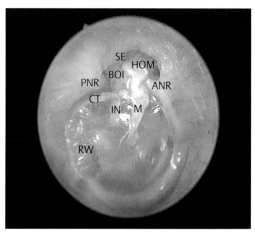

Fig. 7.2.2 Grade II pars flaccida retraction of right ear. Pars flaccida has touched malleus and incus. ANR, anterior notch of Rivinus; BOI, body of incus; CT, chorda tympani; HOM, head of malleus; IN, incus; M, malleus; PNR, posterior notch of Rivinus; RW, round window; SE, scutum erosion.

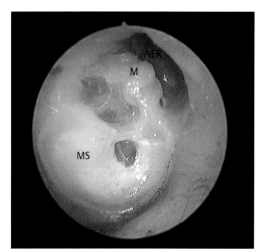

Fig. 7.2.3 Grade III pars flaccida retraction of right ear with definite scutum erosion. Anterior epitympanic recess (AER) is clearly visible through scutum erosion. Malleus head is noticeable, and also one must appreciate myringosclerosis (MS) in pars tensa. M, malleolus.

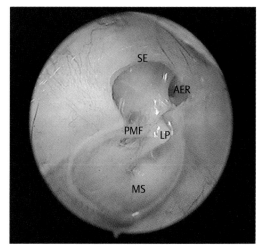

Fig. 7.2.4 Grade III pars flaccida retraction. AER, anterior epitympanic recess; LP, lateral process of malleus; MS, myringosclerosis; PMF, posterior malleolar fold; SE, scutum erosion.

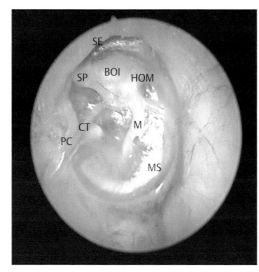

Fig. 7.2.5 Grade IV pars flaccida retraction with scutum erosion going beyond visualization. Head of malleus, body of incus with short process of incus are seen through scutum erosion. Long process of incus is necrosed, chorda tympani (CT) is seen emerging from posterior canaliculus (PC), and myringosclerosis (MS) is noticed in the anterior-inferior part of pars tansa. BOI, body of incus; HOM, head of malleus; M, malleus; SE, scutum erosion; SP, short process of incus.

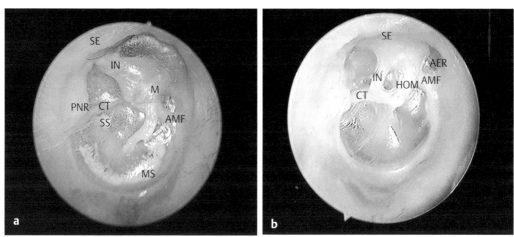

Fig. 7.2.6 **(a)** Grade IV retraction of pars flaccida. In this picture, full malleus and body of incus are visible. Necrosis of lenticular process and diffuse myringosclerosis (MS) are noted. **(b)** Grade IV retraction of pars flaccida of right ear. IN, incus; HOM, head of malleus; M, malleus; MS, myringosclerosis; AER, anterior epitympanic recess; AMF, anterior malleolar fold; CT, chorda tympani; SE, scutum erosion; SS, stapes suprastructure.

7.3 Posterosuperior Retraction Pockets

Though theoretically posterosuperior pockets (PSRP) fall into pars tensa retraction, i.e., inferior-to-posterior malleolar fold, it is commonly accompanied by pars flaccida retraction, cholesteatoma, etc.

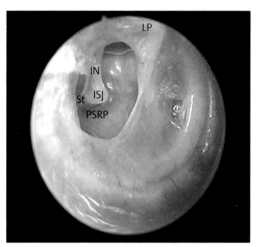

Fig. 7.3.1 Posterosuperior pocket (PSRP) of right ear (LP, lateral process of malleus; IN, incus; ISJ, incudostapedial joint; St, stapedius). One can notice necrosis of lenticular process (may be partial).

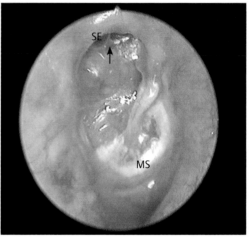

Fig. 7.3.2 Posterosuperior pocket (PSRP) of right ear with grade IV retraction of pars flaccida, incus erosion, and scutum erosion (SE). We cannot determine the extent of retraction pocket. Along with this, there is diffuse myringosclerosis (MS).

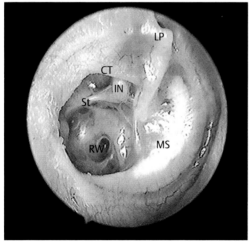

Fig. 7.3.3 A typical posterosuperior pocket (PSRP) of right ear with diffuse myringosclerosis (MS). It is Grade III retraction, where pars tensa has adhered to promontory, round window. CT, chorda tympani; IN, incus; LP, lateral process; MS, myringosclerosis; RW, round window; St, stapedius.

8 Chronic Otitis Media

8.1 Chronic Otitis Media (Mucosal Type)

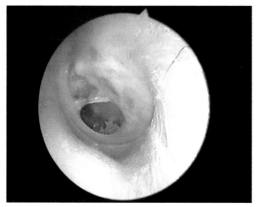

Fig. 8.1.1 Chronic otitis media (mucosal) with moderate central perforation in the anterior-inferior quadrant of pars tensa of left ear.

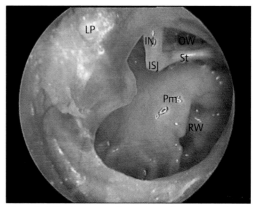

Fig. 8.1.2 Large subtotal perforation of left ear. Different middle ear structures can be well visualized through the perforation. Lateral process (LP), incus (IN), incudostapedial joint (ISJ), stapes suprastructure with stapedius (St), oval window (OW), round window (RW) niche, promontory (Pm) can be visualized clearly. One can notice that there is no residual tympanic membrane in the posterior quadrant.

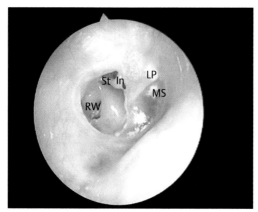

Fig. 8.1.3 Chronic otitis media with large marginal perforation of right ear. Round window (RW), incudostapedial joint, and stapedius (St) are visible through the perforation. Small myringosclerosis (MS) patch is noticed in the anterosuperior quadrant.

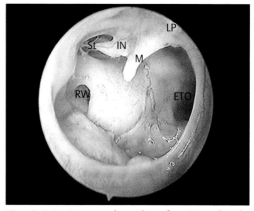

Fig. 8.1.4 Large subtotal perforation of right ear. Eustachian tube orifice (ETO), round window (RW), and stapedius (St) are well seen through the perforation. Foreshortening of malleus is noted here (M, malleus; IN, incus).

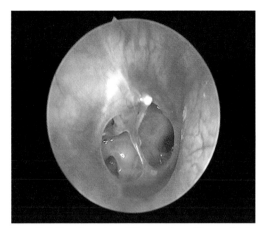

Fig. 8.1.5 Chronic otitis media with multiple perforations of right ear. Two perforations both anterior and posterior to malleus are noticed.

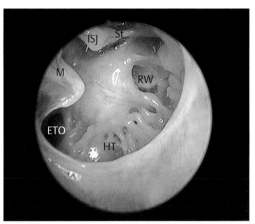

Fig. 8.1.6 Chronic otitis media with large central perforation (CP) of left ear, one can see a kidney-shaped large perforation through which different middle ear structures are seen. Typical irregular bony arrangements are seen in hypotympanum (HT). ETO, Eustachian tube orifice; ISJ, incudostapedial joint; M, malleus; RW, round window; St, stapedius.

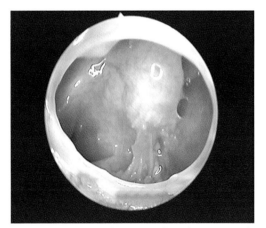

Fig. 8.1.7 Large almost total perforation with discharge is noticed.

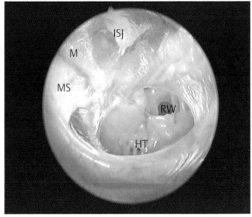

Fig. 8.1.8 Chronic otitis media with central perforation (left ear). Inferiorly placed perforation with myringosclerosis (MS) in the anterosuperior quadrant. Incus and incudostapedial joint (ISJ) are noticed through thinned remnant tympanic membrane, round window (RW), hypotympanum (HT).

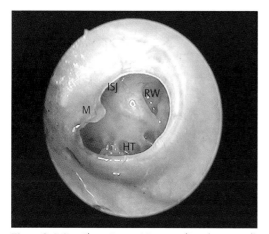

Fig. 8.1.9 Chronic otitis media (mucosal) with large central perforation. Malleus is seen medialized. HT, hypotympanum; ISJ, incudostapedial joint; M, malleus; RW, round window

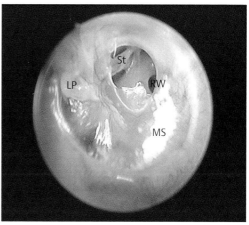

Fig. 8.1.10 Posterosuperior perforation, incudostapedial joint, stapedius, and part of round window are noticed. Diffuse myringosclerosis in posteroinferior quadrant is noticed. LP, lateral process; MS, myringosclerosis; RW, round window; St, stapedius.

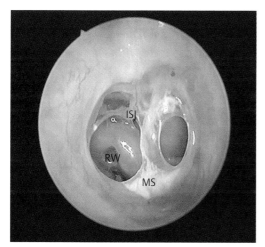

Fig. 8.1.11 Right ear chronic otitis media (mucosal) with multiple perforations. Myringosclerosis patch is located (MS) in between the two perforations. Incudostapedial joint (ISJ) and round window (RW) are seen through posterior perforation.

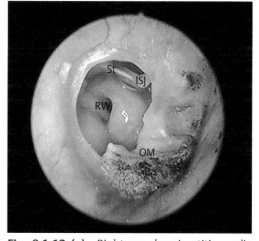

Fig. 8.1.12 (a) Right ear chronic otitis media (mucosal) with posterior perforation and otomycosis (OM) in deep external auditory canal. One can notice incudostapedial joint (ISJ), round window (RW), and stapedius (St) through the perforation.

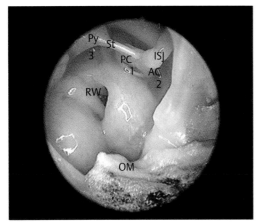

Fig. 8.1.12 (b) A closer look into middle ear through perforation. One can clearly see stapedius (St) originating from pyramid (Py) and inserted into neck of stapes. Anterior crura (AC), posterior crura (PC), and footplate (1) can be seen. Part of oval window niche anterior to anterior crura (AC) is known as fissula ante fenestram (2). Deep sinus tympani (3) are also noticed going beyond pyramidal eminence (sinus tympani grade II type).

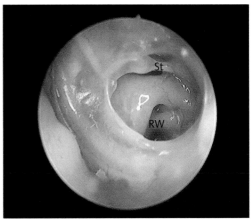

Fig. 8.1.13 Left ear chronic otitis media with posterior perforation. Stapedius (St) and round window (RW) are noticed through perforation.

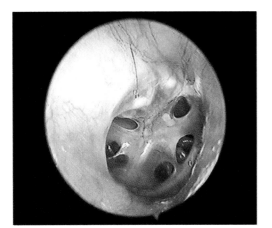

Fig. 8.1.14 Right ear chronic otitis media with multiple perforations. This patient underwent RT-PCR from middle ear fluid and found to be positive for tuberculosis. So it was a case of tuberculous otitis media.

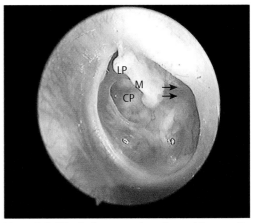

Fig. 8.1.15 Left ear chronic otitis media (mucosal) with grade III retraction of pars tensa (*arrows*) and a perforation at anterosuperior quadrant. CP, central perforation; LP, lateral process; M, malleus.

8.2 Chronic Otitis Media (Squamous type)

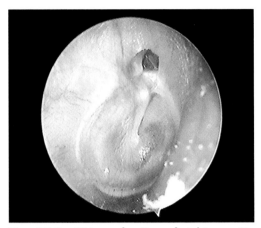

Fig. 8.2.1 Attic perforation of right ear. No frank cholesteatoma is seen.

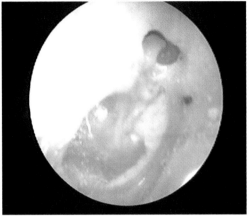

Fig. 8.2.2 Attic retraction with perforation of right ear. Head of malleus is seen through it. Myringosclerosis patch (MS) in the anterosuperior quadrant of pars tensa is noticed. Erosion of outer attic wall is seen.

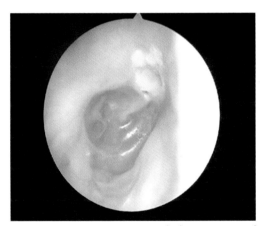

Fig. 8.2.3 Anterior attic cholesteatoma of right ear. Yellowish white cholesteatoma is seen through attic perforation.

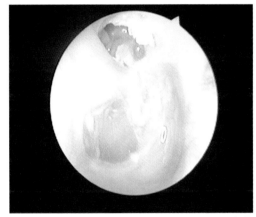

Fig. 8.2.4 Extensive anterior attic cholesteatoma of right ear with definite scutum erosion. Yellowish cholesteatoma is noticed at attic.

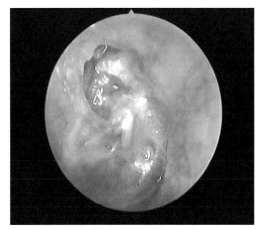

Fig. 8.2.5 Cholesteatoma of right ear in attic with erosion of outer attic wall. Cholesteatoma flakes are noticed through eroded scutum.

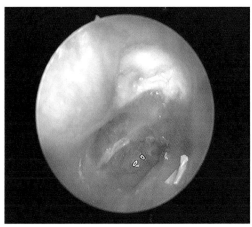

Fig. 8.2.6 Pearly white cholesteatoma in attic region with complete erosion of outer attic wall.

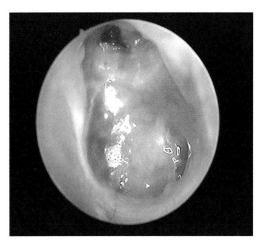

Fig. 8.2.7 Atelectasis of pars tensa with grade IV retraction of pars flaccida and cholesteatoma of right ear. Incus is not visible.

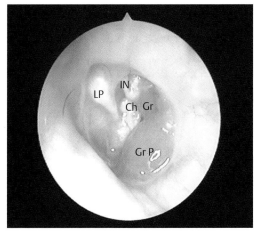

Fig. 8.2.8 Chronic otitis media (squamous) of left ear. Granulation polyp (GP) is seen coming out from sinus tympani region. Mesotympanic cholesteatoma (Ch) is also noticed. Gr, granulation; Gr P, granulation polyp; IN, incus; LP, lateral process.

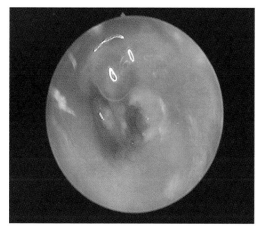

Fig. 8.2.9 Chronic otitis media (squamous) with granulation polyp seen at attic region with cholesteatoma flakes posteriorly.

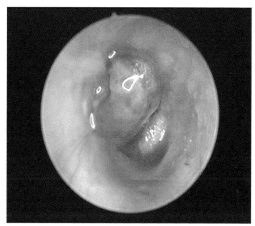

Fig. 8.2.10   A huge granulation polyp from attic and posterosuperior region occupying whole of the tympanic membrane.

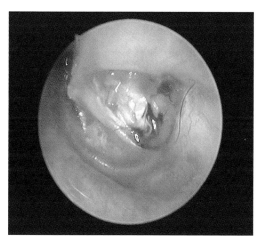

Fig. 8.2.11   Mesotympanic cholesteatoma of left ear. Posterosuperior retraction with cholesteatoma along with anterior attic perforation (AP) with cholesteatoma.

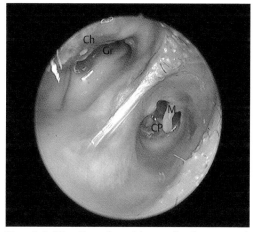

Fig. 8.2.12   Chronic otitis media (squamous) of right ear with central perforation and auto-mastoidectomy. Granulation (Gr), cholesteatoma (Ch), and pus are seen in the automastoidectomy cavity.

9 Tympanosclerosis

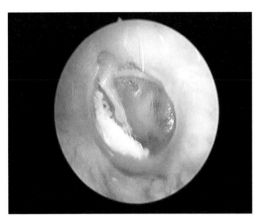

Fig. 9.1 Wooly myringosclerosis in pars tensa of left tympanic membrane at anterior quadrant with intact tympanic membrane.

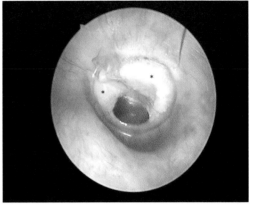

Fig. 9.2 Large myringosclerotic patches anterior and posterior to the handle of malleus are seen. Posterior large myringosclerotic patch extending up to annulus is also seen. In between, there is monomeric tympanic membrane.

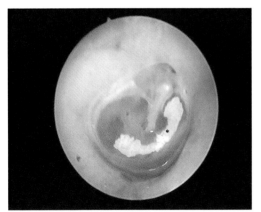

Fig. 9.3 Wooly myringosclerosis patch in intact tympanic membrane.

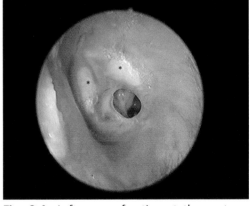

Fig. 9.4 Left ear perforation at the postero-inferior quadrant. Two large myringosclerosis patches are noted at anterior superior and posterior quadrants of pars tensa.

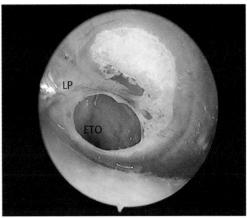

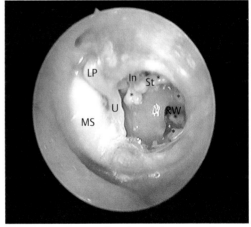

Fig. 9.5 Large perforation of right tympanic membrane with myringosclerosis plaque in the anterosuperior quadrant of pars tensa which is closely adhered to the malleus handle. This type of myringosclerosis is generally accompanied by diffuse tympanosclerosis of middle ear. Malleus incus can be fixed with hard tympanosclerosis of anterior malleolar fold and attic region.

Fig. 9.6 Right ear. Chronic otitis media with central perforation with wooly myringosclerosis patch. This myringosclerosis patch is not extending up to the annulus. ETO, Eustachian tube orifice; LP, lateral process.

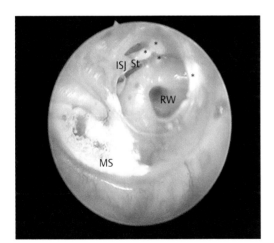

Fig. 9.7 Left ear—posterior marginal perforation, wooly myringosclerosis (MS) at anterior quadrant, and tympanosclerotic patches noted over stapedius and pyramidal process. One can expect ossicular fixation, especially fixation of stapes. ISJ, incudostapedial joint; RW, round window; St, stapedius.

Fig. 9.8 Posteriorly placed large perforation of left ear. Anteriorly crescent-shaped large myringosclerosis patch (MS) adhered to handle of malleus. Diffuse tympanosclerotic patches can be noted in incudostapedial joint (ISJ), stapedius (St), promontory, and round window (RW) region. In this case, we shall find ossicular fixation due to tympanosclerosis. We have to preserve the ossicular integrity while meticulously removing tympanosclerosis. IN, incus; LP, lateral process; RW, round window; St, stapedius; U, umbo.

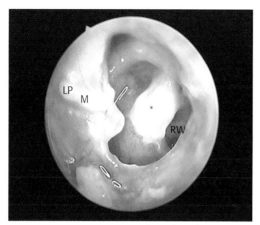

Fig. 9.9 Large posteriorly placed marginal perforation with tympanosclerotic plaque (*asterisk*) over promontory. LP, lateral process; M, malleus; RW, round window.

10 Trauma to the Tympanic Membrane

10.1 Traumatic Perforation

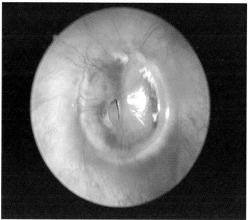

Fig. 10.1.1 Small tiny perforation at the posteroinferior quadrant due to physical trauma to the tympanic membrane. One can notice the blood clot at the anterior margin of perforation.

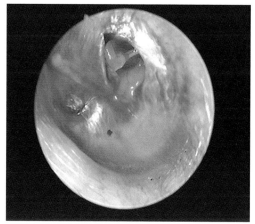

Fig. 10.1.2 Severe physical blow to ear producing posterior perforation with blood in posterior mesotympanum. Margins of perforation are ragged.

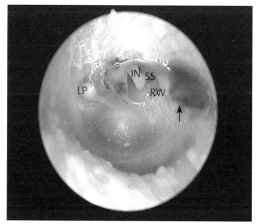

Fig. 10.1.3 Traumatic perforation of left ear. Blood clot is seen in deep external auditory canal. Hemorrhagic spots can be noticed at the margin of perforation, and spots near stapes (SS), incus (IN), and round window (RW) are seen through perforation. LP, lateral process.

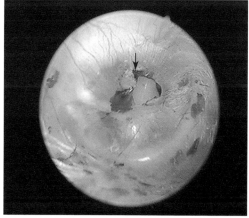

Fig. 10.1.4 Traumatic perforation in healing stage (Day 4 after injury). Blood clots are still in place. These will act as a scaffold upon which neotympanum will grow.

10.2 Barotrauma

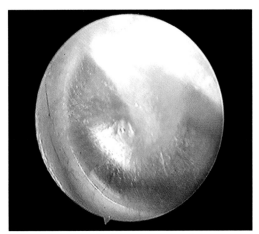

Fig. 10.2.1 Grade I barotrauma with congested pars tensa in anteroinferior quadrant.

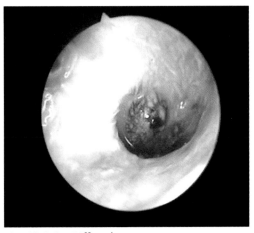

Fig. 10.2.2 Diffuse hemotympanum.

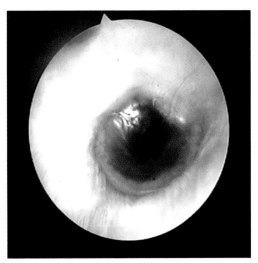

Fig. 10.2.3 Consolidated blood in middle ear 7 days after the incident.

Section B

Surgeries of the Ear

---

11 General Considerations

11.1 Harvesting Temporalis Fascia

Position of the Patient

Supine, head rotated in the opposite direction. Head will rest in a soft head ring; patient should be as close to the surgeon as practicable. Head end should be elevated 10 to 15 degrees. Surgeon is seated comfortably at the side of operation table in a surgeon's stool. Surgeon's back should be straight. Elevate the bed so that there is not much flexion of the neck of the surgeon.

Local Anesthesia

■ Preparation

10 mL of 2% Xylocaine with 1:200,000 adrenaline, 10 mL of distilled water, and 10 drops of 1:1000 adrenaline freshly prepared just before surgery. In case of mastoid surgery, when we operate in general anesthesia, the author infiltrates local anesthesia 10 minutes before incision. Special consideration regarding extra 10 drops of adrenaline should be taken while injecting in old patients or patients with cardiac ailments.

■ Where to Inject

Under proper light, the area two finger breadths above the pinna is infiltrated for harvesting temporalis fascia. Then under microscope, all quadrants of external auditory canal are infiltrated. The author uses 26-gauge needle with 2 mL syringe for this. The bony cartilaginous junction toward the bony side is injected. Injection should be very gentle and slow so that no blebs are formed. Postaural groove, tragus, and incisura terminalis are also infiltrated. After the injection, a cotton pack is put inside the canal for even distribution of the anesthetic agent. Then the scrub nurse will massage this region gently for 5 to 10 minutes. The incision is made after 8 to 10 minutes.

Incisions

■ Postauricular

After proper cross-hatching, an incision is made 5 mm posterior to postaural crease/groove. With proper hemostasis the incision proceeds through posterior auricular muscle, reaching the bone just posterior to Spine of Henle.

■ Endaural Incision/Canal Splitting Incision

At incisura terminalis, medial to lateral incision is made. The lateral meatal flap, i.e., the part of canal lateral to the canal incision, is elevated from medial to lateral direction and held with toothed forceps before putting retractors.

Curvilinear canal incision is made from superior canal wall to posterior and then extended onto anterior canal wall. The ends are 5 mm from annulus whereas the incision in the posterior canal is 10 mm from annulus.

■ Endomeatal Incision

Only canal incision.

Soft Tissue Work

■ Conchotomy Incision

In postaural approach, one has to incise the posterior canal skin at the correct location—if it is done more medially, a small tympanomeatal flap will be created, and if it is done too laterally, a thick flap will be formed; both are difficult to manipulate. Two small release incisions at two margins of conchotomy will help the tympanomeatal flap to settle well onto bony canal wall.

Canalplasty

■ Soft Tissue Canalplasty

To remove the extra soft tissue attached to tympanomeatal flap, make a thin tangential incision at the conchotomy region and remove the deep soft tissue to increase the canal circumference to some extent.

■ Bony Canalplasty

The aim is to view all around the bony annulus—practically the important areas are the anterior canal, inferior canal, and posteroinferior canal. For an anterior wall canal bulge, an incision is made on the bulge and tympanomeatal flap is elevated medial to lateral from the incision. The bulge is then drilled with a diamond burr of an appropriate size. Always protect the medial flap with cotton or aluminum foil. Be careful about not exposing the blue lining of the temporomandibular joint (TMJ).

Drilling of posteroinferior and posterior canal region is tricky. Remember that the vertical part of the facial nerve is few millimeters posterior and medial to the bony annulus in this region.

The aim of canalplasty is to observe the bony annulus in all directions with a single position of the microscope.

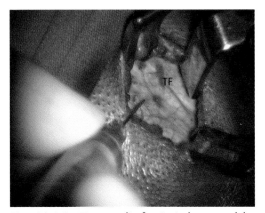

Fig. 11.1.1 Temporalis fascia is harvested by separate incision two finger breadths above the pinna. It can also be harvested from the same postaural or endaural incision. Here hydrodissection is in progress, where normal saline is injected just beneath the temporalis fascia so that it is dissected from the muscle (TF, temporalis fascia).

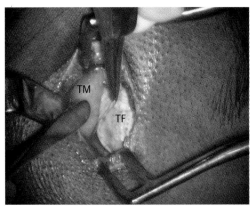

Fig. 11.1.2 Freer's elevator is used to elevate fascia from the temporalis muscle. Temporalis fascia is thick at the insertion of temporalis muscle which is anteroinferior. We have to avoid that part for harvesting (TM, temporalis muscle; TF, temporalis fascia).

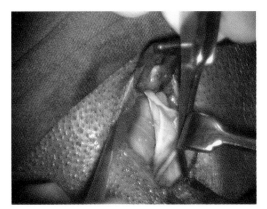

Fig. 11.1.3 Dissection in progress.

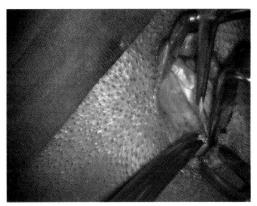

Fig. 11.1.4 Temporalis fascia is harvested by sharp fine scissors, dissecting gently off temporalis muscle. Hemostasis is secured and wound is closed with 3–0 monofilament.

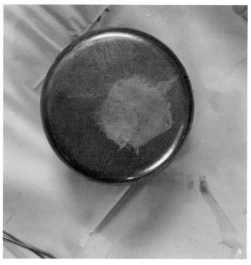

Fig. 11.1.5 Temporalis fascia is spread over the back of a surgical gallipot. Muscle fibers are scrapped out and it is left to dry.

11.2 Incision and General Consideration

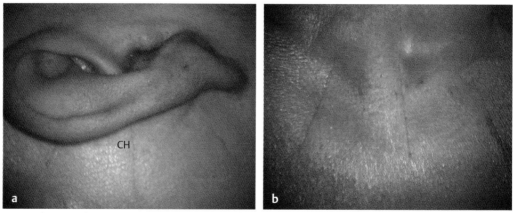

Fig. 11.2.1 (a, b) Right ear postaural incision. Before incision, cross-hatching is done. It is very helpful during suturing and avoids a cosmetic complication called bat ear. CH, cross-hatching.

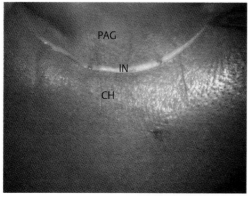

Fig. 11.2.2 Postaural incision is made 5 mm behind the postaural groove. CH, cross-hatching; IN, incision; PAG, postaural groove.

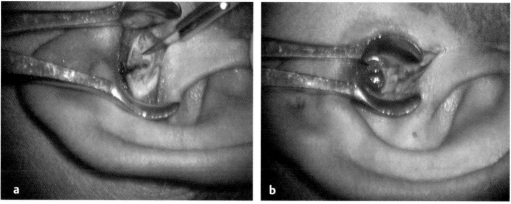

Fig. 11.2.3 (a, b) Endaural incision. Incision in the left ear through incisura terminalis. Lempert's speculum dilates the ear canal and incision is made between the two blades of the speculum.

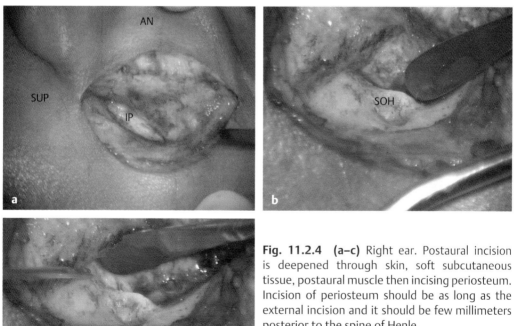

Fig. 11.2.4 (a–c) Right ear. Postaural incision is deepened through skin, soft subcutaneous tissue, postaural muscle then incising periosteum. Incision of periosteum should be as long as the external incision and it should be few millimeters posterior to the spine of Henle.

Periosteum is incised just posterior to the spine of Henle. Now with Freer's elevator dissect canal tissue from the spine of Henle. Gently dissect anteriorly and medially from the spine before performing conchotomy. AN, aterior; IP, incision in periosteum; SOH, spine of Henle; SUP, superior.

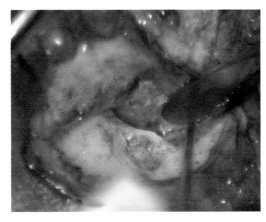

Fig. 11.2.5 Conchotomy incision is made at the level just medial to the spine of Henle. Two release incisions are made at the superior and inferior ends of conchotomy incisions.

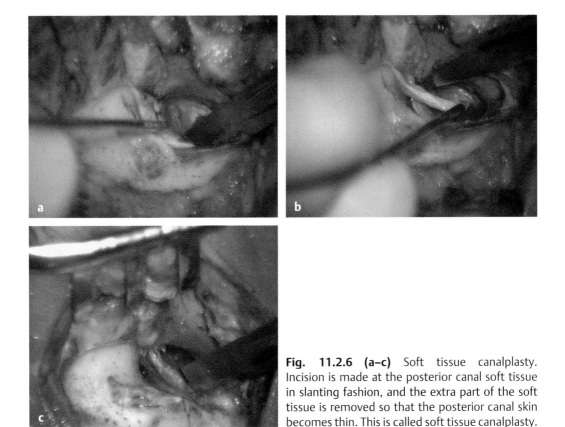

Fig. 11.2.6 (a–c) Soft tissue canalplasty. Incision is made at the posterior canal soft tissue in slanting fashion, and the extra part of the soft tissue is removed so that the posterior canal skin becomes thin. This is called soft tissue canalplasty.

12 Tympanoplasty

Freshening of Margin

The author puts small puncture wounds with needle around the perforation margin and joins them together to remove a thin part of the margin. Scrapping from the undersurface of the remnant of tympanic membrane is done to remove the ingrowth of squamous epithelium.

Tympanomeatal Flap Elevation

For the first few millimeters (medially) near the tympanic membrane, elevate the tympanomeatal (TM) flap medial to lateral. Put the circular knife medial to the TM remnant through perforation at anterior and anterior-inferior quadrant and elevate few millimeters.

Then put two canal incisions: one superiorly with no. 15 blade, meeting the superior edge of the conchotomy incision, and another one inferiorly with circular knife at first at anterior canal starting 5 mm from annulus coming back curvilinear to meet the inferior edge of the conchotomy incision.

After completing the incision, start elevation of the TM flap at the posterior wall, then moving to the superior, inferior, and anterior walls. TM flap is densely adhered to tympanosquamous suture line superiorly and tympanomastoid suture line inferiorly. Here

sharp dissection with no. 15 blade is advisable. It is also advisable to keep adrenaline-soaked Gelfoam at the incision line and to suck onto it, not directly on the flap so that it does not tear.

Elevation of TM Flap

It should continue few mms anterior to the lateral process of the malleus almost up to the anterior notch of Rivinus. Only at the 1 o'clock to 3 o'clock positions (of right ear), TM flap is attached to the canal wall; rest is elevated and tucked anteriorly.

Isthmuses

Always check for any granulation, glue, or diseased mucosa near ossicles. For that curette or drill the posterosuperior quadrant and place an adrenaline-soaked Gelfoam at this area and then gently remove the diseased mucosa by small right-angled pick. During this procedure, always keep the orientation of mucosal fold in your mind. After clearing all granulation and glue from the posterosuperior quadrant, check the ossicular mobility. For that, put a curved needle just beneath the lateral process of malleus and gently push medially; one can notice the movement of all ossicles. Similarly, gentle push on the long process of the incus to appreciate the movement of stapes and footplate.

If any ossicle is necrosed, do the required ossiculoplasty (see "Ossiculoplasty").

Placing the Graft

After carefully inspecting ossicles, middle ear mucosa, place the graft on the canal bone except the anterosuperior part where the TM flap is attached to the canal wall.

Here the graft will be tucked under the annulus. Repose the TM flap and place dry Gelfoam at anterior sulcus. This will hold the graft and TM flap while maneuvering the graft.

Again the graft with TM flap is elevated and ciprofloxacin-soaked Gelfoam is placed in the middle ear, especially the anterosuperior quadrant anterior to the malleus.

Now, both TM flap and graft are repositioned and under higher magnification all quadrants are visualized for perfect contact between graft and perforation margin.

Placing of Gelfoam

Small pieces of ciprofloxacin-soaked Gelfoam are placed after removing the dry Gelfoam which was placed before. The author puts Gelfoam first anterosuperiorly, then all along the perforation margin coming up to the canal incision point. In most of the cases, he does not put any pack, but sometimes gives Neosporin H-soaked ribbon pack at the end; wound is closed with 3–0 monofilament suture in single layer, and mastoid dressing is done.

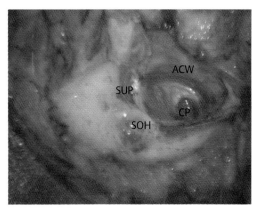

Fig. 12.1 Right ear. Central perforation (CP) at the anteroinferior quadrant seen after conchotomy and soft tissue canalplasty. ACW, anterior canal wall; SOH, spine of Henle; SUP, superior.

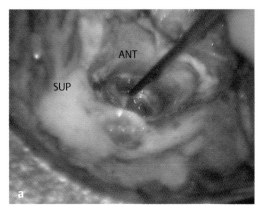

Fig. 12.2 (a) Incision at anterior canal wall with circular knife starting at 1 o'clock position 5 mm from the remnant of tympanic membrane. (ANT, anterior; SUP, superior.

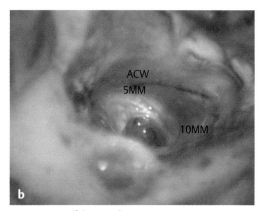

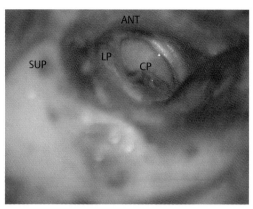

Fig. 12.2 (b) Curvilinear incision at anterior canal wall starting at the 1 o'clock position then going laterally about 10 mm at inferior and posterior walls then communicating with conchotomy incision. ACW, anterior canal wall.

Fig. 12.3 Freshening of margin. Multiple perforations are made with needle along the rim of perforation then they are joined together to remove the margin of perforation. ANT, anterior; CP, central perforation; LP, lateral process; SUP, superior.

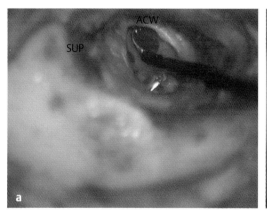

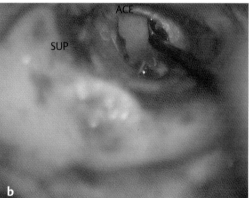

Fig. 12.4 (a, b) Removing squamous epithelium from the undersurface of the perforation. The author elevates few mms of tympanomeatal flap putting the circular knife medial to the perforation. This is done at the anterior canal only. ACW, anterior canal wall; SUP, superior.

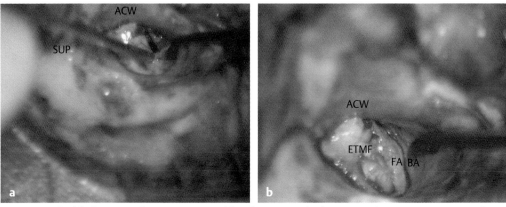

Fig. 12.5 **(a, b)** Elevation of tympanomeatal flap from 11 o'clock position (posterosuperior quadrant) to 1 o'clock position (anterosuperior quadrant) is done with circular knife and suction. You can notice fibrous annulus (FA) and bony annulus (BA) at the anterior canal wall. ACW, anterior canal wall; ETMF, elevated TM flap.

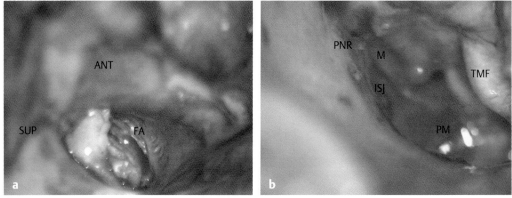

Fig. 12.6 **(a, b)** Medial mucosal layer of tympanic membrane is incised between fibrous annulus (FA) and bony annulus anteriorly and in posterosuperior quadrant where bony annulus is missing. ANT, anterior; ISJ, incudostapedial joint; M, malleus; PM, promontory; PNR, posterior notch of Rivinus; SUP, superior; TMF, tympanomeatal flap.

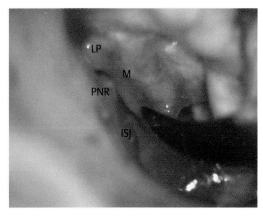

Fig. 12.7 Incision on the malleus with sickle knife is made to denude the malleus. ISJ, incudostapedial joint; LP, lateral process; M, malleus; PNR, posterior notch of Rivinus.

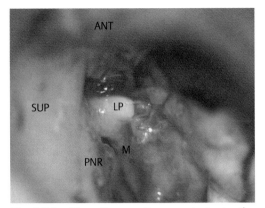

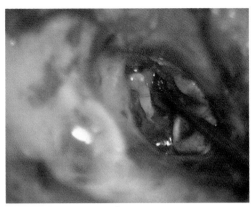

Fig. 12.8 Dissection continues anterior to the lateral process (LP); with the back of sickle knife tympanomeatal flap is dissected anteriorly. M, malleus; PNR, posterior notch of Rivinus.

Fig. 12.9 Anterior dissection continues up to the 1 o'clock position. This anterior to malleus dissection is a very important step to place the fascia anterosuperior to the malleus directly on the bony canal.

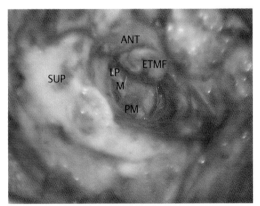

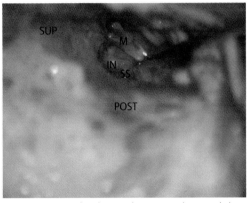

Fig. 12.10 After complete elevation of tympanomeatal flap, it is tucked anterosuperiorly. Almost 300 degrees (from 1 o'clock to 11 o'clock position) of bony canal is bare and temporalis fascia can rest over the bare bony canal and can get its nutrition from it. This helps in complete graft uptake. ANT, anterior; ETMF, elevated TM flap; LP, lateral process; M, malleus; PM, promontory.

Fig. 12.11 Checking the ossicular mobility. Drilling of posterosuperior quadrant was carried out. Put curved needle just beneath the lateral process and gently push the malleus medially to check whether ossicles are moving or not. IN, incus; M, malleus; POST, posterior; SS, stapes suprastructure; SUP, superior.

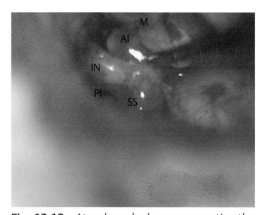

Fig. 12.12 At a closer look, one can notice the anterior isthmus (between malleus and incus) and posterior isthmus (posterior to incus). Small pick over lenticular process and incudostapedial joint and gentle push medially will produce movement of stapes and footplate. AI, anterior isthmus; IN, incus; M, malleus; PI, posterior isthmus; SS, stapes suprastructure.

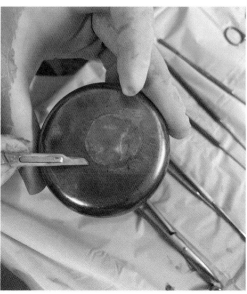

Fig. 12.13 Temporalis fascia is gently elevated from the back of the bowl with no. 15 blade.

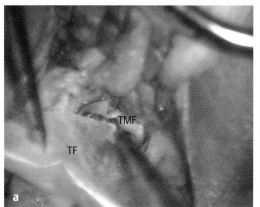

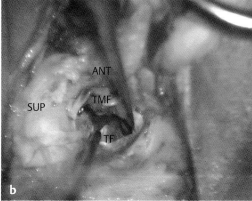

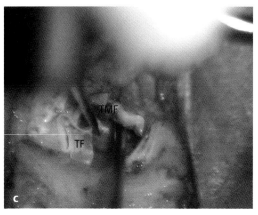

Fig. 12.14 **(a–c)** Hold the temporalis fascia with alligator and gently push forward toward the anterior wall and spread the fascia with needle simultaneously. ANT, anterior; SUP, superior; TF, temporalis fascia; TMF, tympanomeatal flap.

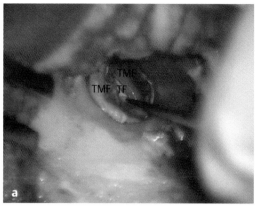

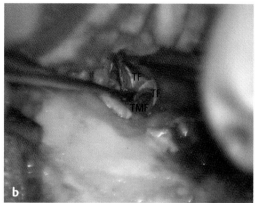

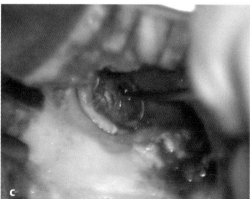

Fig. 12.15 **(a)** After proper placement of fascia onto bony canal, the tympanomeatal flap is placed over it. Here one can see the temporalis fascia (TF) through the perforation after proper placement of tympanomeatal flap (TMF). **(b)** Anteriorly TMF is again elevated and one can see TF under it all along. One can see that temporalis fascia is placed over the canal bone all along the canal (here anterior, anteroinferior, posteriorly). **(c)** Again temporalis fascia along with TM flap is repositioned. Anterior fibrous annulus is secured at the exact point of bony annulus.

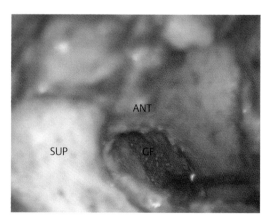

Fig. 12.16 A dry Gelfoam (GF) is placed at the anterior sulcus to hold the fibrous annulus at the exact position. ANT, anterior; SUP, superior.

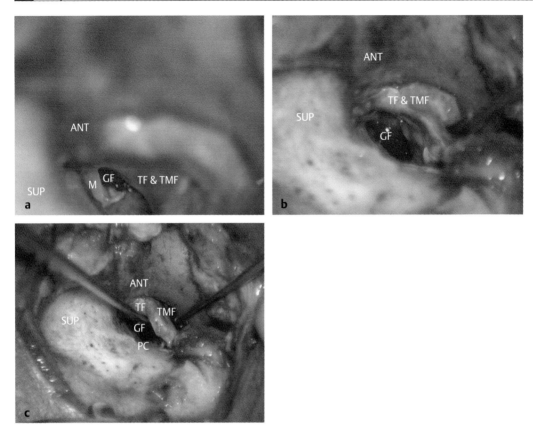

Fig. 12.17 **(a)** Placement of Gelfoam in middle ear. Tympanomeatal flap (TMF) and temporalis fascia (TF) is elevated anteriorly and Gelfoam (GF) is placed anterosuperiorly to malleus first. **(b)** Few Gelfoams are placed in middle ear for providing support to TF from the middle ear side. **(c)** Now TF and TMF are repositioned. Here, the author uses a repositor in the right hand to be placed onto TF and needle in the left hand is placed under TMF. Then repositor is gently pushed towards the bony posterior canal while the needle keeps the lateral part of TF away from posterior canal. This maneuver helps to remove air trapped in the middle ear. ANT, anterior; M, malleus; PC, posterior canal; SUP, superior).

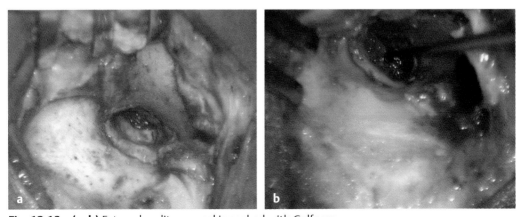

Fig. 12.18 **(a, b)** External auditory canal is packed with Gelfoam.

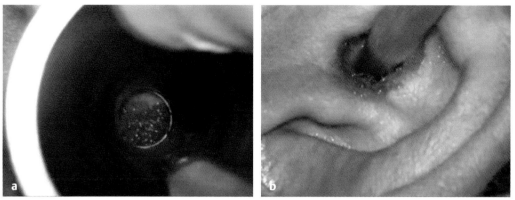

Fig. 12.19 (a, b) After placing Gelfoam up to canal incision, aural speculum is placed and rotated gently so that canal skin is unrolled and spread over the graft. Few Gelfoams are placed in the canal.

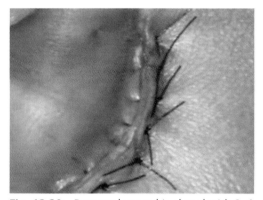

Fig. 12.20 Postaural wound is closed with 3–0 monofilament in a single layer.

13 Ossiculoplasty

Decision Making

A number of options are available for ossiculoplasty, including cartilage, reshaped ossicles, and prosthesis of different types. Different factors like the ossicular status (whether stapes suprastructure is present or not) and materials available for reconstruction and skill required for it determine the type of ossiculoplasty. One has to be conversant with all techniques before conducting this surgery.

Important Terminologies

- **Partial prosthesis:** Prosthesis onto intact stapes suprastructure.
- **Total prosthesis:** Prosthesis onto mobile footplate when stapes suprastructure is absent.
- **Short columella of cartilage:** Onto intact stapes head.
- **Long columella of cartilage:** Onto mobile footplate.

Incus Necrosis

Long process/Lenticular process of incus: partial necrosis.

a) Necrosis <10% (visual assumption): one can wrap the incudostapedial joint (ISJ) and lower part of the long process of the incus with periosteum.

b) Necrosis >10% or if fibrous band at ISJ region: take out incus, then plan ossiculoplasty, either cartilage short columella, reshaped autoincus short columella, or partial ossicular prosthesis (POP).

- **Options:** Reshaping of incus for transposition over stapes suprastructure as short columella.
- Interposition is done between malleus and stapes suprastructure; interposition technique is difficult and provides same result as of transposition technique.
- **Preserved cartilage short columella:** Short columella with hole for stapes head at one side. The height of columella should not be beyond neoannulus after putting it over stapes suprastructure.
- **Prosthesis:** POP with cartilage cap so that prosthesis does not come in direct contact with neotympanum. The author sutures the thin-sliced cartilage with titanium plate using 6–0 Vicryl.

Stapes Suprastructure Necrosis

The author uses only three options:

1. Cartilage long columella from preserved cartilage. Pointed end of the columella should be onto footplate and extended end will touch the neotympanum. The height of the columella should not be more than neoannulus.

2. If malleus is salvageable, then malleus can be reshaped and used as long columella. Here, the author cuts the malleus just above the lateral process and reverses its orientation placing pointed end onto footplate.

3. Titanium total prosthesis with cartilage shoe and cartilage cap so that prosthesis does not touch footplate and neotympanum directly. Cartilage shoe can be made from thin-sliced cartilage and its size will be same as a 26-gauge suction tip. Cartilage cap is sutured with titanium plate using 6–0 Vicryl.

A tricky situation arises when stapes head, neck, part of anterior crura, and part of posterior crura are missing. The author tends to do fancy cartilage reshaping to resemble absent stapes suprastructure. But in his experience, he has observed that the long-term hearing outcome of this type of assembly is not good. For him, simple cartilage long columella from footplate (between anterior crura and posterior crura) to neotympanum is the best option.

In the review of the study regarding the results of different types of ossiculoplasty, we inferred that:

- Presence of stapes suprastructure is the single most important factor for good hearing outcome.

- Percentage of extrusion of prosthesis (Polytetrafluroethylene (PTFE) or titanium) is significantly higher.

- Incus interposition between malleus and stapes is technically challenging and yields no higher results than incus-short columella (transposition).

- Cartilage short columella provides same or better long-term result than costly prosthesis.

- Cartilage long columella provides definitely better result than total prosthesis.

In this context, the author defines good hearing outcome if pure tone average is less than 20 dB and there is air bone gap less than 20 dB. If the difference of pure tone audiometry (PTA) between two ears is less than 30 dB, patient senses better hearing.

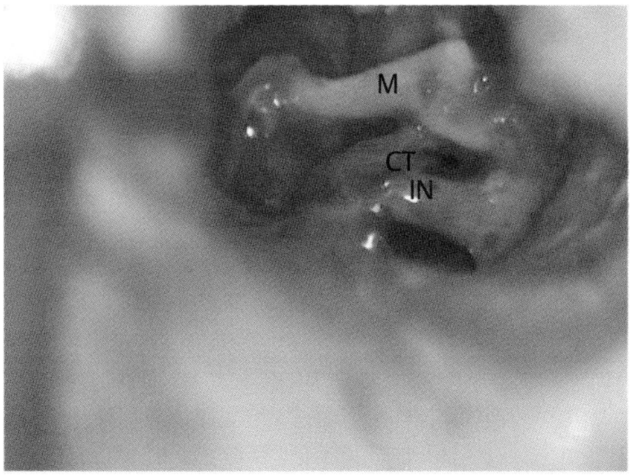

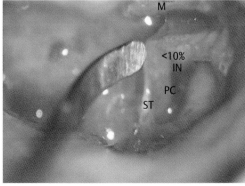

Fig. 13.1 Posterosuperior quadrant drilling. (Left ear). After removal of posterosuperior bony canal wall, one can visualize malleus (M), Incus (IN), Chorda tympani (CT) nerve, and posteromesotympanum.

Fig. 13.2 (Left ear) incus-partial necrosis <10%. M, malleus; IN, incus; PC, posterior crura of stapes; ST, stapedius tendon.

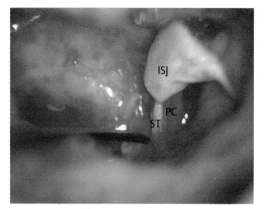

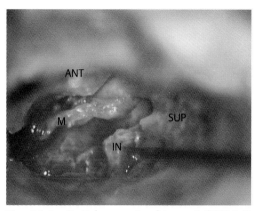

Fig. 13.3 In this case, long process of incus, incudostapedial joint (ISJ) is covered with periosteum, and this assembly works fine. PC, posterior crura of stapes; ST, stapedius tendon.

Fig. 13.4 Partial necrosis of incus (>75%) left ear. In this case, incus is removed and cartilage short columella assembly is performed. ANT, anterior; IN, incus; M, malleus; SUP, superior.

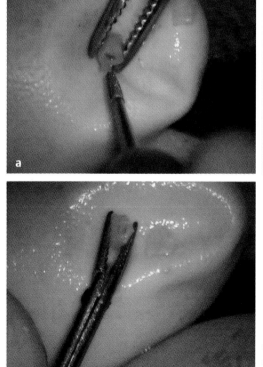

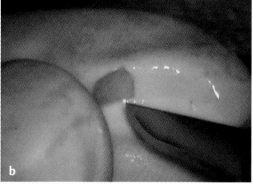

Fig. 13.5 (a–c) Process of making short columella. Small strut of preserved nasal septal cartilage is modified and small hole for stapes head is made with dental burr.

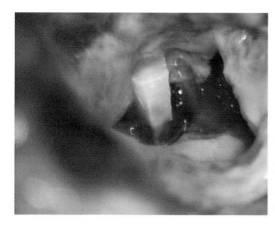

Fig. 13.6 Cartilage short columella is placed over stapes head and supported with Gelfoam. The height of columella should not be more than annulus. Short columella will increase the middle ear space and provide good hearing.

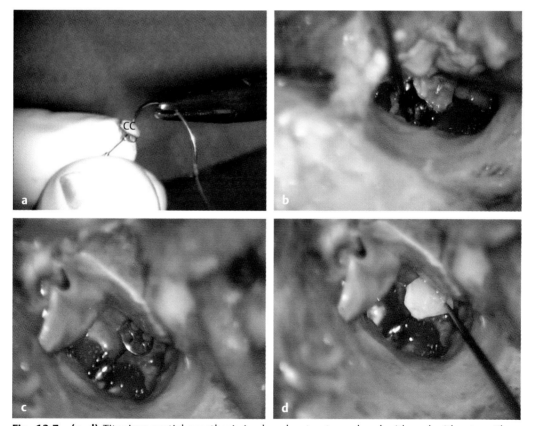

Fig. 13.7　(a–d) Titanium partial prosthesis is placed onto stapes head with and without cartilage cap (CC). The author sutures the cartilage cap with prosthesis using 6–0 Vicryl. Cartilage cap helps to prevent extrusion of prosthesis, although the author has found that the percentage of extrusion of prosthesis is relatively high.

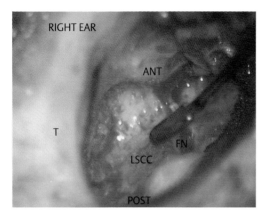

Fig. 13.8 Stapes suprastructure is missing; footplate is in place and mobile. Here one can notice lateral semicircular canal (LSCC) fistula, dehiscent facial nerve (FN). ANT, anterior; POST, posterior; T, tegmen.

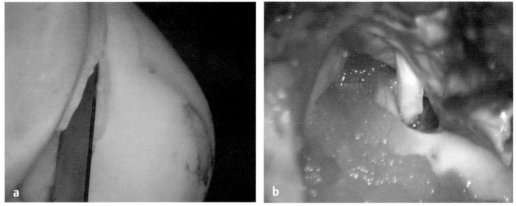

Fig. 13.9 **(a, b)** Making of long columella. A vertical strut is created from preserved nasal septal spur cartilage. One tip is sharp and pointed, which will be placed on footplate, and the other will touch neotympanum. Here long columella is placed on foot plate and is supported with Gelfoam.

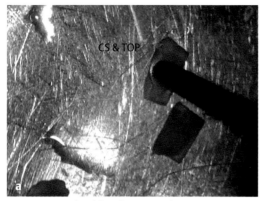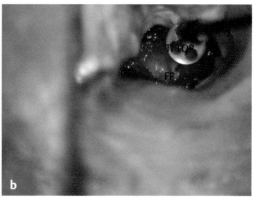

Fig. 13.10 **(a, b)** When we place titanium total prosthesis, we put cartilage shoe medially and cartilage cap laterally. For cartilage shoe, a thin-sliced cartilage is cut in the same size of a 26-gauge suction tip and placed medially onto the shaft. It is placed onto footplate and supported by Gelfoam and soft tissue. Here titanium (Ti) total prosthesis with cartilage shoe is placed onto mobile footplate (right ear) after that cartilage cap will be placed so that there will be no direct contact between prosthesis and neotympanum which reduces the chance of extrusion of prosthesis. CS, cartilage shoe; FP, stapes footplate; TOP, prosthesis.

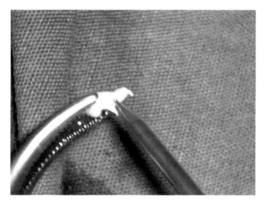

Fig. 13.11 Sculpturing of autoincus. Incus is held with forceps and sculpturing is done with a 0.6-mm diamond burr.

14 Mastoid Exploration

Decision Making

Do not be preoccupied by the approach, i.e., inside-out or outside-in before seeing the pathology.

The approach should suit pathology. Here the author shall discuss the way he approaches mastoid disease. There are different approaches. All lead to the same goal: total clearance of disease, preservation of hearing, and reconstruction of cavity. One must learn each approach but practice the approach that suits best in his/her hand. One must execute same approach repeatedly and become master of that.

In mastoid exploration surgery, our goal is:

1. Complete disease clearance.
2. Reconstruction of hearing as far as practicable.
3. Cavity reconstruction.

Finer Aspects

- Position of the patient.
- Infiltration of local anesthesia.
- Incision: Postaural.
- Soft tissue dissection: Curvilinear incision along postaural groove near the spine of Henle. Put a horizontal incision along the lower border of temporalis muscle and elevate periosteum in all directions.

- Elevation of tympanomeatal (TM) flap without conchotomy from the spine of Henle up to few mms lateral to annulus.
- Sharp conchotomy incision is made more medially (near the annulus) than that of tympanoplasty.
- Ribbon gauze is passed through external ear and taken out through conchotomy; this will act as anterior retractor.
- 3/4 hook self-retaining retractors are placed.
- Rest of tympanomeatal flap along with tympanic membrane is elevated and placed anteriorly.
- Cover foil of catgut suture is cut into small pieces placed over TM flap to protect it from rotating drill.
- Here, always try to preserve chorda tympani nerve. If it is not possible, try to cut it with scissors sharply keeping few mms as it emerges from posterior canaliculus. This will act as a surgical landmark while drilling posterosuperior quadrant.

Removal of Disease

- Start drilling with large conical burr and ask the assistant to put water slowly drop by drop so that bone dust from the cortical bone accumulates. Then collect it with Freer's elevator put at the edge of a bowl, and instill few drops of ciprofloxacin ear drop in it. Let it dry.

- Take a comparatively bigger burr and start drilling in the posterosuperior quadrant, attic, and anterior attic region. One can see malleus head, incus body, etc., if present at this stage.

- If incus is necrosed, remove it. Follow the disease posteriorly up to sinodural angle. Remove each bit of cholesteatoma and granulation from dural plate, sinus plate, and sinodural angle region.

- Sometimes dural breach is noticed. If you can do high-resolution computed tomography (HRCT) temporal bone before mastoid surgery, you can see and predict the dural breach before even seeing it. Dural breach should be anticipated beforehand. The dural plate is anteriorly sloped, i.e., the height reduces as it approaches middle ear; this anatomy should always be kept in mind.

  ◇ If there is granulation tissue over intact dura, one can remove it with bipolar cautery.

  ◇ In case of small dural breach with no cerebrospinal fluid (CSF) otorrhea, it need not be closed. But if it is >1 cm, it can be covered with fascia and a slice of cartilage.

- In case of CSF otorrhea, first try to locate the site of leak, then close it in three layers—fascia, cartilage, fascia. The author uses bipolar to make dural surface a bit raw then puts fascia under the bony breach covering raw dura. Next, he insinuates a thin-sliced cartilage (few mms bigger than bony breach) between fascia and the bony defect, and finally, again a layer of fascia on the top of it. This robust assembly is supported by Surgicel and even muscle patch or temporalis muscle pedicled flap.

- Clearing of sinodural region is very important as it is a place for residual disease, and sinodural angle should be opened as wide as possible. Small bits of granulation tissue should be removed with diamond drill under higher magnification.

- Clearing sinus plate is another important step. Drilling with large diamond burr while approaching sinus plate is an important trick to avoid sinus penetration. If you can do HRCT temporal bone before surgery, you can anticipate sinus dehiscence beforehand. Sometimes if granulation tissue is adhered to dehiscent sinus wall, then sinus rupture can occur. Do not panic. Put a large piece of gauze pack and keep pressure and in the meantime arrange for Surgicel. Do not give small pieces of AbGel inside the open sinus. Take a long piece of Surgicel and put one end inside the sinus and the other end between the bone and sinus wall and wait for some time. Put gauze pack over it and wait for few more minutes. Bleeding will stop. Now, proceed to other areas.

- Now deal with facial ridge. It is the bone of posterior and inferior wall of external auditory canal lying lateral to vertical facial nerve. The author drills it with a large diamond burr, to lower the facial ridge. At this point, he thins the ridge along with lowering it. Drilling should continue in the deep external canal near annulus so that facial recess and hypotympanum will be opened up. One must keep in mind that facial nerve elevates only few mms from second genu to stylomastoid foramen. Another landmark is lateral semicircular canal (LSCC); facial nerve lies anterior and medial to LSCC at second genu region. Keeping these landmarks in mind, facial ridge is lowered so that middle ear and mastoid cavity become a single cavity.

- Now our attention is shifted toward LSCC. Sometimes fistula is noted in LSCC. Fistula test can provoke vertigo or dizziness and nystagmus in LSCC fistula patient. HRCT can pick up it before surgery. Granulation tissue or cholesteatoma around or above fistula is peeled off gently along with copious irrigation with Ringer Lactate solution. This step should be done at the end of the procedure. After removal of disease, one can see whether endosteal layer is intact or not. It should be covered by fascia and cartilage. The author puts bone dust around it so that fistula is covered adequately.

- From our very beginning years, we have been taught about facial palsy as the dreaded complication of mastoid surgery. It has created a dogma in our mind. But believe the author, facial nerve is our friend and guide, not foe. It is one of the more consistent landmarks in mastoid surgery. Dehiscence of facial nerve in the horizontal part and second genu is pretty common. Granulation over the horizontal part of facial nerve has to be dissected with blunt instrument with great caution. Processus cochleariformis acts as guide to horizontal facial nerve. Sometimes granulation tissue adheres with vertical facial nerves intimately. Here also dissection should be along the course of the facial nerve with great caution under higher magnification.

- Dealing with ossicles is a very important step in mastoid surgery. The author tries to preserve malleus head as far as possible to maintain a scaffold for attic reconstruction. Sometimes when the disease goes medial to malleus head then the malleus head has to be removed. One can cut the tensor tympani at processus cochleariformis and rotate malleus laterally to gain access to the medial to ossicles.

  ◇ If incus is necrosed >10 to 15% at lenticular process, it is better to remove it. Then, plan ossiculoplasty accordingly at the end stage of surgery.

- Granulation tissue over stapes has to be dissected from posterior to anterior direction. One has to remember different mucosal folds around stapes during this step. After removal of disease there will be two situations—either stapes-suprastructure present or not. We have to plan ossiculoplasty depending on the situation.

- Removal of disease from facial recess and sinus tympani is an important step to reduce the chance of residual disease. While thinning facial ridge, the lateral wall of facial recess is removed, giving full access to these regions. In case of very deep (Grade II/III) sinus tympani, angled otoendoscope may help.

- After complete removal of disease, the author uses a large diamond burr to polish the bony edges so that there is no sharp angulation and cavity becomes smooth.

Reconstruction of Hearing

See the section on ossiculoplasty.

Cavity Reconstruction

- First conchomeatoplasty—It is a very important step for future surveillance and thereby reducing the chance of recurrence. The author follows a simple technique. First, a vertical incision through external auditory meatus toward concha for few mms. Then, dissect out conchal cartilage from meatus side.

  Now from postaural side "T"-shaped incision is made meeting the previous incision. Removal of inferior external auditory canal cartilage (which is thick) is very important to reduce the recoil of cartilage. Then, suture both flaps, everting the skin with Vicryl/catgut. It is sutured inferiorly to the soft tissue near the tip and superiorly to the temporalis muscle. Thus, nicely skin-lined, adequate-sized meatoplasty is created.

- Reducing the depth of cavity by bone dust in sinodural angle, tip area, or other areas of deep crevices.

- Then layer of cartilage harvested from conchomeatoplasty incision is placed over bone dust to maintain the height of attic region.

- Graft is placed over it and TM flap is repositioned over it and a large piece of dry Gelfoam is placed at anterior annulus region. Next, fascia graft and TM flap are elevated again, and ossiculoplasty is done. Middle ear is gently packed with ciprofloxacin-soaked small pieces of Gelfoam. Graft and TM flap are repositioned.

- Muscle pedicle flap: Posteriorly or anteriorly based half-thickness temporalis muscle pedicle flap is elevated and placed onto the graft. In my series, I found this step is very useful to reduce the cavity size and to give almost normal looking cavity afterwards.

- Few pieces of antibiotic-soaked Gelfoam are given over this muscle graft–TM flap. At the end, ear is packed with bismuth iodoform paraffin paste (BIPP) soaked roller gauze pack and wound is closed with 3–0 monofilament.

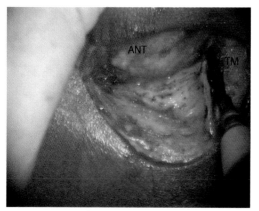

Fig. 14.1 Left ear mastoid exploration. Curvilinear incision of periosteum and horizontal incision of periosteum at the temporal line. ANT, anterior; TM, temporalis muscle.

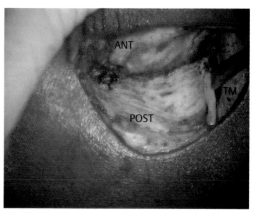

Fig. 14.2 Periosteum elevator is used to elevate temporalis muscle and posterior auricular muscle. ANT, anterior; POST, posterior; TM, temporalis muscle.

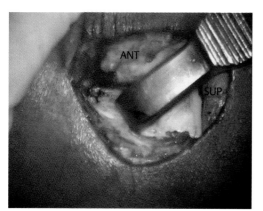

Fig. 14.3 Farabeuf's periosteal elevator is used to elevate posterior musculoperiosteal flap. ANT, anterior; SUP, superior.

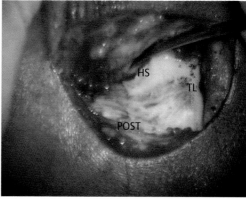

Fig. 14.4 Now using Freer's elevator, posterior canal skin is elevated from the posterior canal bone starting from the spine of Henle (HS). Here, elevation should go to the superior canal wall and posteroinferior canal wall. One should go medially up to annulus in case of mastoid exploration so that large amount of posterior canal skin is preserved. POST, posterior; TL, temporal line.

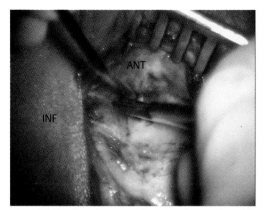

Fig. 14.5 Conchotomy incision is made with knife as medially as possible near the annulus. ANT, anterior; INF, inferior.

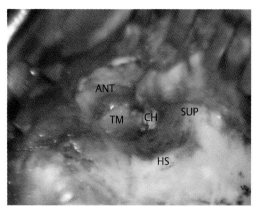

Fig. 14.6 After conchotomy incision is complete, self-retaining mastoid retractors are placed. One can see cholesteatoma (CH) at attic region and intact pars tensa tympanic membrane (TM), spine of Henle (HS). ANT, anterior; SUP, superior; TM, tympanic membrane.

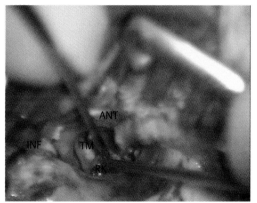

Fig. 14.7 Deep canal skin (only few mms medial to conchotomy incision) is elevated with round knife (RK) and suction. ANT, anterior; INF, inferior; TM, tympanic membrane.

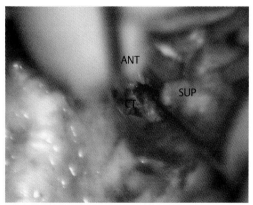

Fig. 14.8 Sharp dissection at posterosuperior quadrant to expose chorda tympani (CT) and the author will try to preserve it. ANT, anterior; SUP, superior.

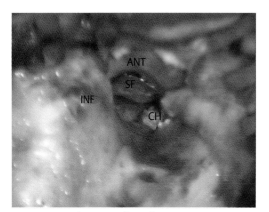

Fig. 14.9 After complete dissection, intact pars tensa is tucked anteriorly and protected with suture foil (SF). It is an important step to protect tympanic membrane from rotating burrs during drilling. ANT, anterior; CH, cholesteatoma; INF, inferior.

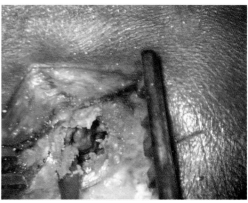

Fig. 14.10 Drilling started on the cortical bone. Bone dust is collected with Freer's elevator and kept at the side of a bowl.

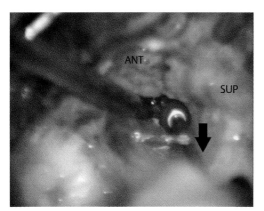

Fig. 14.11 After canalplasty, a large cutting burr is used to drill posterosuperior bony wall near annulus. This inside-out drilling is done in medial to lateral fashion. ANT, anterior; SUP, superior.

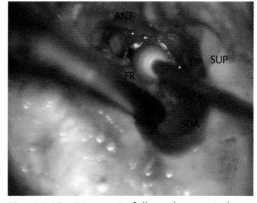

Fig. 14.12 Disease is followed posteriorly up to sinodural angle (SDA) region. Superiorly dural plate (DP) is delineated and a large diamond burr is used to drill the facial ridge (FR). ANT, anterior; SDA, sinodural angle; SUP, superior.

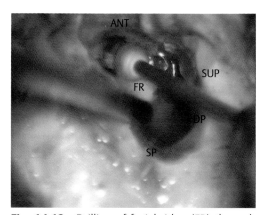

Fig. 14.13　Drilling of facial ridge (FR) through canal side is carried out. It is known as thinning of facial ridge. This step also opens the facial recess and sinus tympani. ANT, anterior; DP, dural plate; SP, sinus plate; SUP, superior.

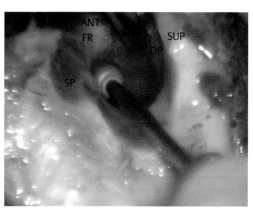

Fig. 14.14　Drilling undersurface of sinus plate (SP). Note the color change of sinus plate region. This is a bit forward lying sinus. Sometimes, diseased mucosa or granulation is noticed undersurface of sinus plate and sinodural region. ANT, anterior; DP, dural plate; FR, facial ridge; SUP, superior).

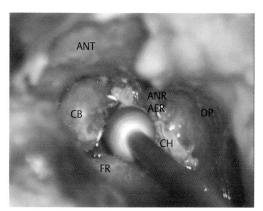

Fig. 14.15　Further drilling of facial ridge (FR) to open up sinus tympani region. Cotton ball (CB) is used to dissect cholesteatoma (CH) from medial wall. Anterior epitympanic recess (AER) is cleared from cholesteatoma. Anterior notch of Rivinus (ANR) is noticed. ANT, anterior; CB, cotton ball; CH, cholesteatoma; DP, dural plate.

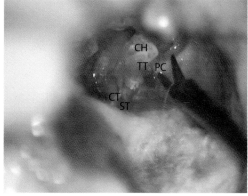

Fig. 14.16　Cholesteatoma is dissected. Tensor tympani (TT) is cut at processus cochleariformis (PC) so that malleus which was entangled inside the matrix can be removed. CH, cholesteatoma; CT, chorda tympani; ST, sinus tympani.

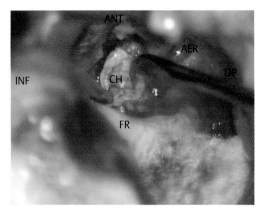

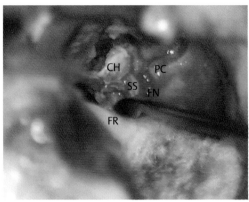

Fig. 14.17 Further dissection with sickle knife removing cholesteatoma (CH) off suprastructure of stapes. AER, anterior epitympanic recess; ANT, anterior; DP, dural plate; FR, facial ridge; INF, inferior.

Fig. 14.18 Stapes suprastructure (SS) is now visible. Cholesteatoma (CH) is gently peeled off from SS. FN, horizontal facial nerve; FR, facial ridge; PC, processus cochleariformis.

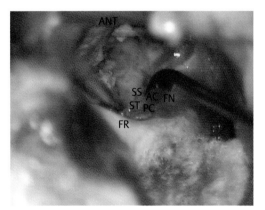

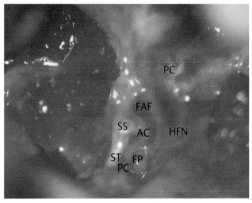

Fig. 14.19 Cholesteatoma is removed. One can notice clearly stapedius (St), posterior crura (PC), anterior crura (AC), stapes head, horizontal facial nerve (FN), facial ridge (FR).

Fig. 14.20 A closer view of stapes. One can see footplate (FP), stapedius (ST), posterior crura (PC), anterior crura (AC), horizontal facial nerve (HFN), processus cochleariformis (PC), and fissula ante fenestrum (FAF).

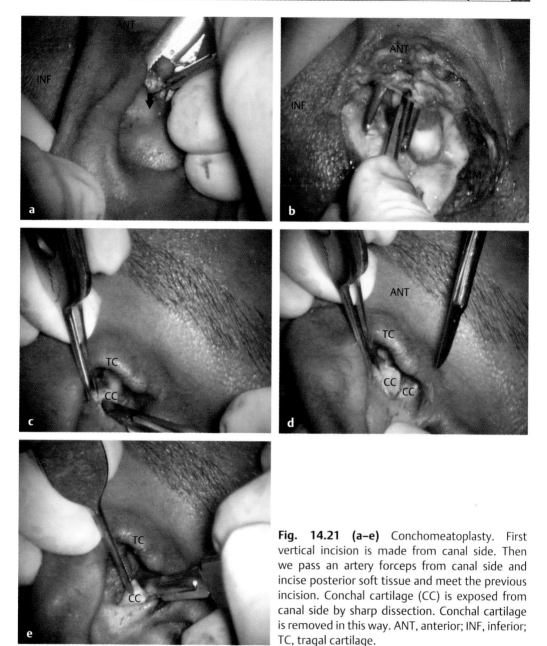

Fig. 14.21 (a–e) Conchomeatoplasty. First vertical incision is made from canal side. Then we pass an artery forceps from canal side and incise posterior soft tissue and meet the previous incision. Conchal cartilage (CC) is exposed from canal side by sharp dissection. Conchal cartilage is removed in this way. ANT, anterior; INF, inferior; TC, tragal cartilage.

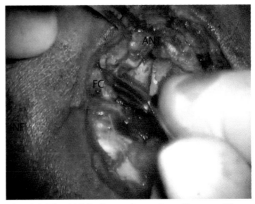

Fig. 14.22 Now from posterior side, two flaps—inferior meatal flap (IMF) and superior meatal flap (SMF)—are created. ANT, anterior; INF, inferior.

Fig. 14.23 With sharp dissection, floor cartilage (FC) of cartilaginous external canal is excised and removed. This is an important step to decrease the recoil of this cartilage. This step prevents narrowing of meatus in future. ANT, anterior.

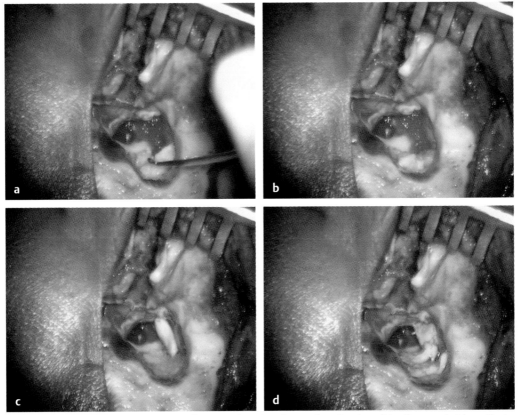

Fig. 14.24 **(a–d)** Reconstruction of mastoid cavity. Bone dust is placed in the mastoid cavity to reduce the size of cavity. Then a layer of cartilage harvested from conchal region is placed over it. Placement of cartilage is done to maintain the height of attic and also in the sinodural angle and sinus plate region.

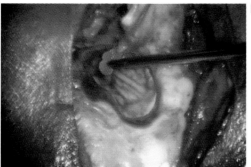

Fig. 14.25   Graft placement.

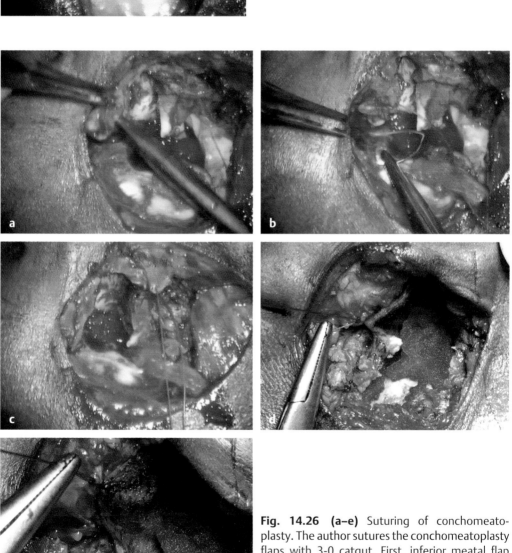

Fig. 14.26 (a–e) Suturing of conchomeato-plasty. The author sutures the conchomeatoplasty flaps with 3-0 catgut. First, inferior meatal flap is secured with the soft tissue near tip region. Superior meatal flap is sutured with temporalis muscle. Skin from the canal is sutured with the soft tissue so that canal skin is everted and lined conchomeatoplasty.

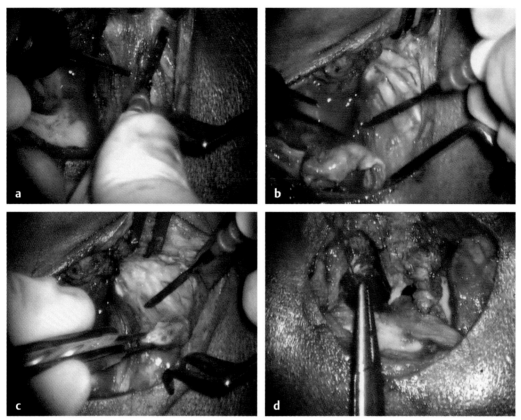

Fig. 14.27 (a–d) Creation of posterior based split thickness temporalis muscle flap was done to obliterate the mastoid cavity. Half thickness temporalis muscle is elevated and rotated keeping a posterior base. Half thickness of temporalis muscle is retained at its original space to prevent hollowing of supra auricular region.

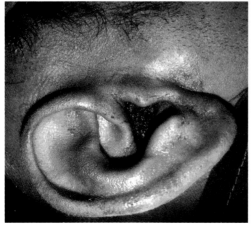

Fig. 14.28 End result of adequate conchomeatoplasty. Conchomeatoplasty should be adequate for the resultant cavity.

14.1 Special Situations

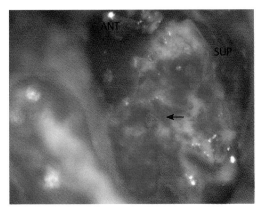

Fig. 14.1.1 Mastoid exploration. Small fistula in lateral semicircular canal (*arrow*) can be noticed. ANT, anterior; SUP, superior.

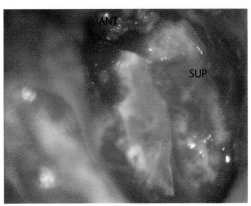

Fig. 14.1.2 Covering lateral semicircular canal (LSCC) fistula first with small piece of fascia. ANT, anterior; SUP, superior.

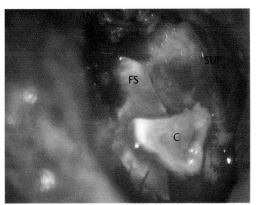

Fig. 14.1.3 Then it is reinforced with cartilage with perichondrium. ANT, anterior; C, cartilage; FS, fascia; SUP, superior.

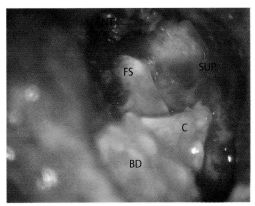

Fig. 14.1.4 Supported with bone dust. ANT, anterior; BD, bone dust; C, cartilage; FS, fascia; SUP, superior.

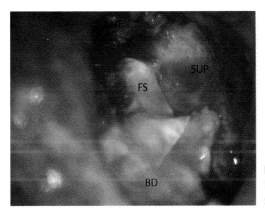

Fig. 14.1.5 Lastly again a fascia on the top of it. (ANT, anterior; BD, bone dust; FS, fascia; SUp, superior).

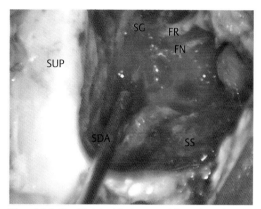

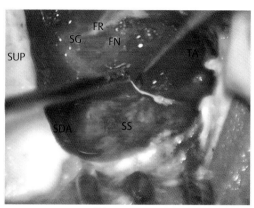

Fig. 14.1.6 Right-sided mastoid exploration in a complicated squamous COM patient with long-standing facial palsy. Entire length of sigmoid sinus (SS) is dehiscent. Vertical part of facial nerve (FN) is exposed inferior to facial ridge (FR) (SDA, sinudural angle; Sup, superior; SG, second genu of facial nerve).

Fig. 14.1.7 Small bits of cholesteatoma matrix is gently peeled off from dehiscent sigmoid sinus (SS) FN, dehiscent facial nerve (vertical part); FR, facial ridge; SDA, sinudural angle; SG, second Genu of facial nerve; TA, tip area.

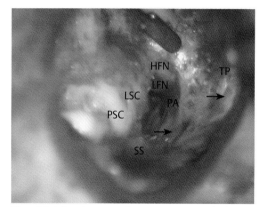

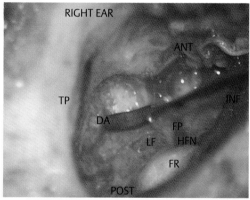

Fig. 14.1.8 A case of petrous apex choleste-atoma (left ear). After complete removal of cholesteatoma one can see dehiscent sigmoid sinus (SS), horizontal facial nerve (HFN) turning on itself at 1st genu and forming labyrinthine facial nerve (LFN). There are also dehiscent lateral semicircular canal (LSC) and posterior semicircular canal (PSC). Tegmen plate (TP) is eroded at different (*arrows*) sites. PA, petrous apex.

Fig. 14.1.9 Right mastoid exploration. Dural dehiscence is noticed in tegmen plate (TP) region; lateral semicircular canal (LSCC) fistula (LF); stapes suprastructure is absent so footplate (FP) is visible; dehiscent horizontal facial (HFN) nerve is also noticed. ANT, anterior; DA, dural dehiscence; FR, facial ridge; INF, inferior; POST, posterior.

15 Stapes Surgery

Decision Making

Age of the patient: If age of the patient is less than 15 years, suspect pathology other than otosclerosis. If age is more than 60 to 65 years, guarded prognosis in hearing gain should be discussed.

Hearing loss: Tuning fork test; BC > AC (bone conduction is better than air conduction) is the most important criteria. Surgery is indicated if pure tone auditory (PTA) is pure conductive or mixed hearing loss with major conductive component. The surgery is contraindicated in pure sensorineural hearing loss (SNHL) or mixed hearing loss (MHL) with major sensory component.

Large air-bone gap corresponds to the amount of footplate fixation. Amount of SNHL corresponds to the amount of cochlear involvement.

Speech discrimination score (SDS): Low SDS is a contraindication for surgery as hearing gain will not be satisfactory after surgery.

Informed Consent

Always mention other options of treatment, i.e., hearing aid. One must definitely discuss the percentage of hearing improvement, chance of permanent hearing loss, percent of vertigo and facial palsy as postoperative complications. Surgeon should mention that this surgery is for hearing improvement, not for improvement of tinnitus in the consent form.

Endaural Incision

Generally, the author prefers endaural or canal splitting incision, and then, puts self-retaining endaural speculum.

Canal Incision

The canal incision is same as that of tympanoplasty but not extended in anterior canal wall. For right ear, incision is given at the 1 o'clock to 5 o'clock positions, at the midpart 10 mm away from annulus and at the extremities going up to 5 mm to annulus. Anterior extension of the incision is anterior to malleus, keeping in mind the rare possibility of malleus-incus ankylosis. Inferiorly, the incision extends up to the round window.

Elevation of TM Flap

Gently elevate TM flap with the help of circular knife and adrenaline-soaked Gelfoam. It should be done simultaneously in all areas. Then reach annulus and gently lift middle ear mucosa.

Entering the Middle Ear

Gently with sickle/needle enter into middle ear by making small nick at mucosal layer and then extending it superiorly and inferiorly. Put 4% Xylocaine-soaked Gelfoam in middle ear for some time.

Managing the Chorda Tympani Nerve

During opening of middle ear space, proper dissection and preservation of chorda tympani nerve is important. The author has noticed that injury to this nerve in chronic ear disease did not produce change of taste but in otosclerotic cases it causes much discomfort. Nevertheless, in some rare cases where space is very little, one has to sharply cut this nerve to gain access.

Checking Ossicular Mobility

After elevation of TM Flap, malleus should not be denuded; putting a needle just below lateral process and gentle medial push will produce malleus-incus movement. Now gently push near lenticular process of incus and see whether any movement of footplate is there or not.

Posterosuperior Bony Overhang

Posterosuperior bony overhang should be either drilled or curetted out.

The author prefers to do it with House curette. Movement of curette should be from medial to lateral and upside down. Small bits of bone should be removed at a time. Removing large chunks should be avoided. Extent of removal should be such that one can visualize part of the long process and

horizontal facial nerve superiorly, and base of pyramid posteriorly.

This step can also be done with drill, skeeter, etc. Extreme caution should be taken so that the curette does not touch the incus while removing the bone. It may cause hypermobile incus.

Measurement

A measuring rod is placed over the footplate. Observe which spike is at the undersurface of the long process of the incus. Before surgery, measure the distance between distant spike and measuring spikes with slide caliper so that exact measurement can be noticed. Now add 0.5 mm (0.25 mm—thickness of footplate +0.25 mm into endolymph) with measured length for the exact length of piston. Take Polytetrafluroethylene (PTFE)/Teflon piston into measuring and piston cutting jig and cut with new no. 15 blade sharply. Now put a curved needle through the loop of piston and dilate it.

Control Fenestra

Now do a control fenestra with 0.3-mm stapes perforator at the posterior part of footplate. Hold the perforator between the thumb and index finger; do not touch the long process of the incus while doing this step. Put the perforator tip onto footplate and gently rotate the perforator between the thumb and index finger. Sudden loss of resistance will mark the opening of footplate.

Gradually increase the size of fenestra by putting 0.5, 0.6-mm stapes perforator through the fenestra. In all these steps, do not give pressure on the footplate.

Now hold the piston at its loop with piston-holding forceps, with both lying at almost at the same line or an angle of 135 degrees.

Gently push the lower end of the piston through fenestra and simultaneously slip the loop around the long process of the incus. Now with crimping forceps, crimp the loop of prosthesis gently.

Disarticulation of Incudostapedial Joint

Incudostapedial joint (ISJ) is disarticulated with sharp joint knife or right-angled sharp pick, entering the joint through the side of promontory, i.e., inferiorly.

First, gently remove a mucosal cover then enter the joint, and with slicing movement, disarticulate ISJ.

Cutting the Stapedius

Stapedius is cut with scissors near the origin at pyramid.

Cutting the Posterior, Anterior Crura

With small, sharp right-angled pick, posterior crura is cut near its base and same is applied to anterior crura. As anterior crura is thin, it is easily broken. Now the entire stapes suprastructure is pushed toward promontory and gently taken out with a forceps.

Small fat from ear lobule harvested early and washed with normal saline is kept near fenestra. Reposition the TM flap and put small pieces of ciprofloxacin-soaked Gelfoam lateral to TM. Wound is closed with 3–0 monofilament.

Stapedectomy

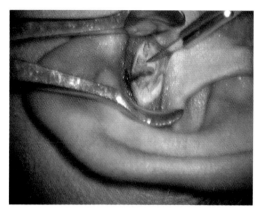

Fig. 15.1 Left ear—endaural incision is in progress through incisura terminalis.

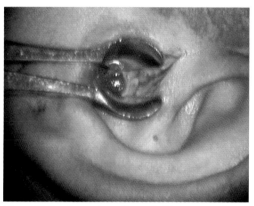

Fig. 15.2 An adrenaline Gelfoam is placed in deep external auditory canal so that blood from endaural incision does not reach tympanic membrane.

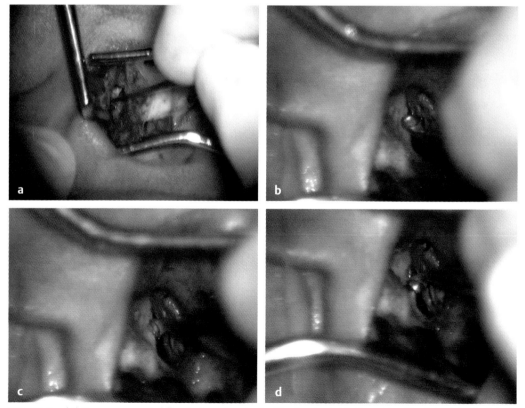

Fig. 15.3 **(a)** Tympanomeatal flap being elevated with circular knife from the 11 o'clock to 5 o'clock position. **(b–d)** Posterosuperior bony overhang is curetted with House curette. The movement of curette is always away from ossicles. This step should be done cautiously so that the curette does not touch the incus which may give rise to hypermobile incus.

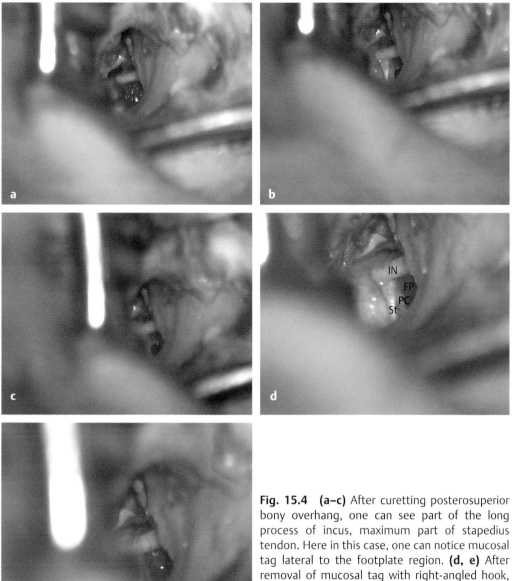

Fig. 15.4 **(a–c)** After curetting posterosuperior bony overhang, one can see part of the long process of incus, maximum part of stapedius tendon. Here in this case, one can notice mucosal tag lateral to the footplate region. **(d, e)** After removal of mucosal tag with right-angled hook, one can clearly see the posterior crura (PC), footplate (FP), stapedius (St), and long process of incus (IN).

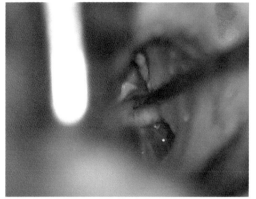

Fig. 15.5 Checking the mobility of stapes, with right-angled pick. By gently palpating over long process of incus, there is no movement of footplate.

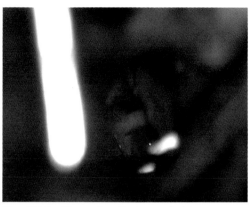

Fig. 15.6 Measuring jig is needed to measure the distance between the undersurface of long process of incus and the footplate. In this case, it was 4 mm. So piston of 4.5 mm will be used.

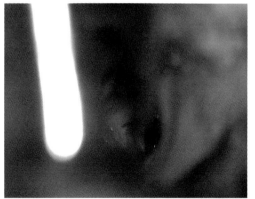

Fig. 15.7 Footplate perforator of 0.3 mm is used to make control hole in the posterior half of footplate. Gradually, the size of fenestra is increased by 0.4-, 0.5-, and 0.6-mm perforator. The shaft of perforator is held by thumb and index finger and perforation is made through gentle rotatory movements.

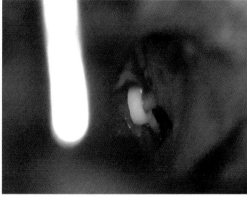

Fig. 15.8 A 4.5-mm stapes piston is placed through fenestra and hooked onto the long process of incus.

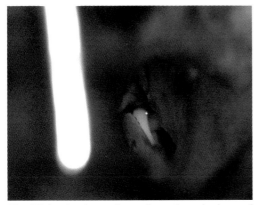

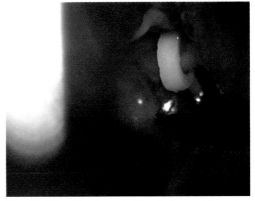

Fig. 15.9 A crimper is used to crimp the loop of piston. It is done neither too hard nor too loosely.

Fig. 15.10 Right-angled hook is used to enter incudostapedial joint from inferior aspect and disarticulate it.

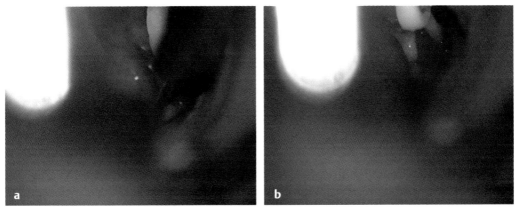

Fig. 15.11   (a, b) A crurotomy scissor is used to cut the stapedius tendon. Stapedius tendon is cut at its base.

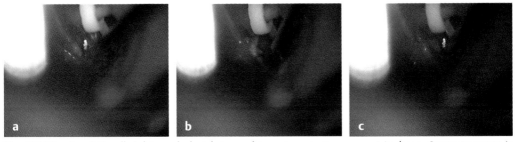

Fig. 15.12   (a–c) Small right-angled pick is used to cut posterior crura at its base. Suprastructure is fractured by pushing it inferiorly toward promontory. Suprastructure is removed.

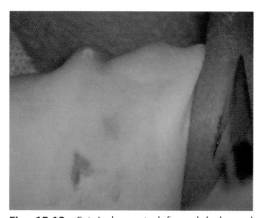

Fig. 15.13 Fat is harvested from lobule and washed in normal saline.

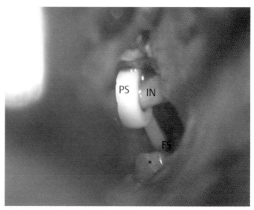

Fig. 15.14 Fat (*asterisk*) is placed posterior to piston near fenestra. FS, fenestra; IN, incus; PS, piston.

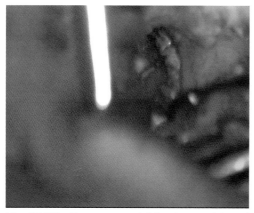

Fig. 15.15 Tympanomeatal flap is repositioned with repositor.

Another Case of Stapedectomy

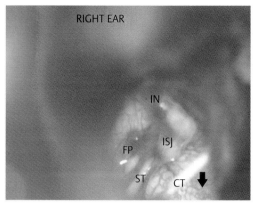

Fig. 15.16 After proper exposure, one can see ISJ (incudostapedial joint), incus (IN), stapedius (ST), footplate (FP), and chorda tympani (CT) here; notice the engorged blood vessels at promontory (*arrow*), which when seen through intact tympanic membrane is known as "Schwartz sign."

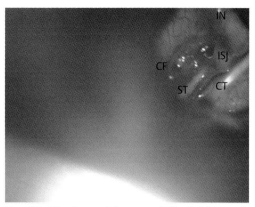

Fig. 15.17 Control fenestra (CF) of 0.3 mm is made with 0.3-mm perforator at the posterior half of footplate. CT, chorda tympani; IN, incus; ISJ, incudostapedial joint; ST, stapedius.

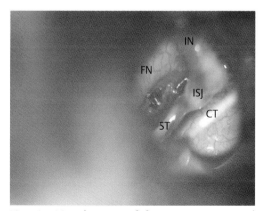

Fig. 15.18 The size of fenestra is increased by 0.4-, 0.5-, 0.6-mm perforator gradually. CT, chorda tympani; FN, facial nerve; IN, incus; ISJ, incudostapedial joint; ST, stapedius.

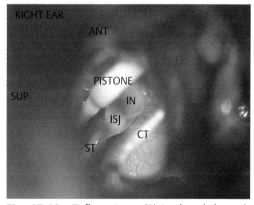

Fig. 15.19 Teflon piston (P) is placed through fenestra and loop is hooked around long process of incus (IN). CT, chorda tympani; ISJ, incudostapedial joint; ST, stapedius.

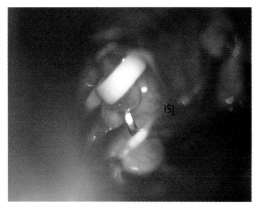

Fig. 15.20 Right-angled hook is used to disarticulate incudostapedial joint (ISJ). The joint is entered from the side of promontory.

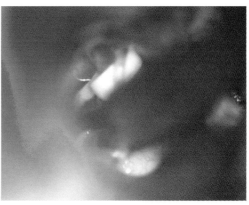

Fig. 15.21 Stapedius tendon is cut with scissors.

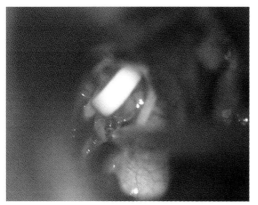

Fig. 15.22 Posterior crura is cut with right-angled pick just above the footplate. Anterior crura is thinner and can be fractured easily.

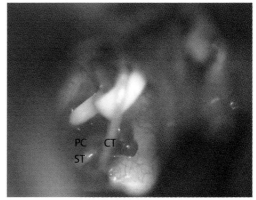

Fig. 15.23 Stapes suprastructure (SS) is fractured toward promontory. CT, chorda tympani; PC, posterior crura; ST, stapedius.

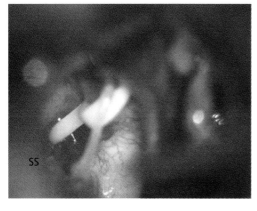

Fig. 15.24 After removal of stapes suprastructure (SS), one can notice that piston is well inside the fenestra and loop is hooked around long process of incus. Chorda tympani is anchored lateral to piston. After that tympanomeatal flap is repositioned and Gelfoam is placed in the auditory canal.

Section C

Radiology of the Ear

16. CT Scan of Temporal Bone in Relation to Chronic Otitis Media (Squamous)

16 CT Scan of Temporal Bone in Relation to Chronic Otitis Media (Squamous)

Aniket Mondal

High-resolution computed tomography (HRCT) of temporal bone has a valuable role in preoperative evaluation of chronic otomastoiditis, providing excellent delineation of the extent of the disease especially in the hidden areas (e.g., sinus tympani and facial recess) as well as the various complications such as bone erosion, ossicular erosion, facial canal erosion, labyrinthine fistula, sigmoid plate dehiscence and erosion of tegmen, and any intracranial extension. In addition, it provides a presurgical roadmap to the surgeon by detecting any anatomical variants (e.g., high riding or dehiscence jugular bulb, dehiscence facial canal, and low lying tegmen) that may lead to life-threatening consequences during surgery. Another important role of computed tomography (CT) is detection of recurrent/residual disease to avoid unnecessary second-look surgical exploration. In this chapter, we have shown different types of disease extent of chronic otomastoiditis especially the cholesteatoma, and its various complications, along with few important anatomical variants.

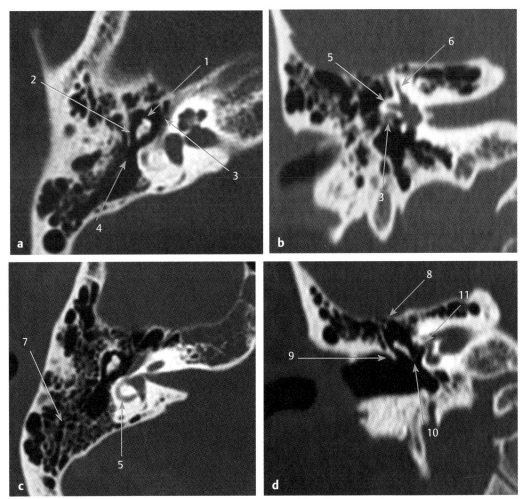

Fig. 16.1 HRCT temporal bone of axial **(a, c)** and coronal **(b, d)** section show normal middle ear and mastoid anatomy. 1: Malleus head, 2: Incus, 3: Facial canal (tympanic segment), 4: Aditus ad antrum, 5: Lateral Semicircular canal, 6: Superior semicircular canal, 7: Mastoid air cells 8: Tegmen, 9: Scutum, 10: Lentiform process of Incus, 11: Stapes in oval window.

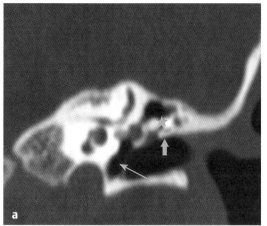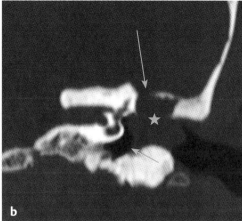

Fig. 16.2 **(a)** Right-sided chronic otitis media—coronal high-resolution computed tomography (HRCT) shows nondependent hypodense soft tissue opacification in Prussak's space (*asterisk*) and epitympanum with erosion of scutum (*thick arrow*)—suggestive of pars flaccida cholesteatoma. **(b)** In addition to this, there is erosion of tegmen antrum (*long thin arrow*) and ear ossicles. Mildly thickened retracted tympanic membrane (*short thin arrow*).

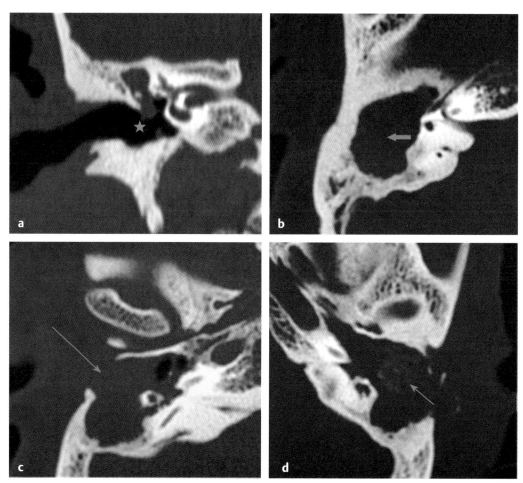

Fig. 16.3 Right-sided chronic otitis media (COM). **(a)** Thickened tympanic membrane with a large central perforation (*asterisk*). **(b, c)** Widening of aditus antrum with erosion of mastoid trabeculae and ear ossicles with formation of common cavity (*thick arrow*). **(c)** In another patient, erosion of lateral wall of mastoid with subperiosteal abscess formation (*long arrow*) leading to automastoidectomy. **(d)** Left-sided COM—automastoidectomy with fibro-osseous changes (*short arrow*) within.

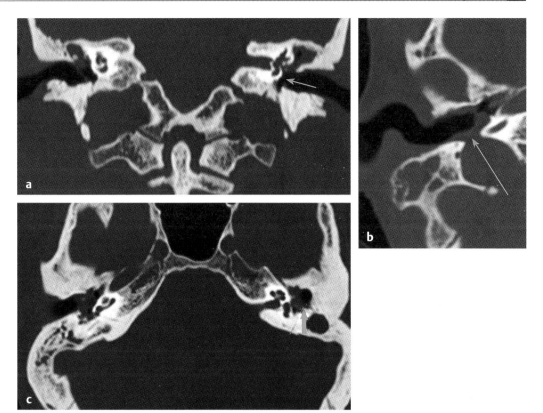

Fig. 16.4   **(a)** Coronal and **(b)** axial—shows bilateral cholesteatoma with marked retraction of tympanic membrane (*short arrow*). Granulation tissue extends into the hypotympanum with dehiscence jugular bulb (*long arrow*) and thick retracted tympanic membrane. **(c)** Granulation tissue involves the sinus tympani and facial recess (*thick arrow*). Figure C is from another patient.

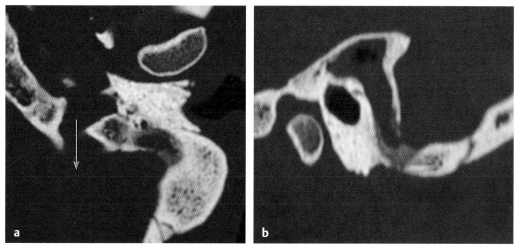

Fig. 16.5 **(a)** Axial and **(b)** sagittal. Left-sided chronic otitis media—focal irregular erosion is seen in sinodural plate (*arrow*).

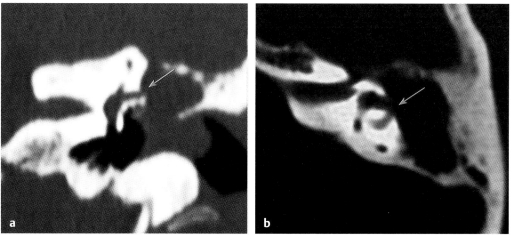

Fig. 16.6 Right-sided chronic otitis media. Coronal **(a)** and axial **(b)** scans show erosion of lateral semicircular canal with formation of labyrinthine fistula (*arrow*).

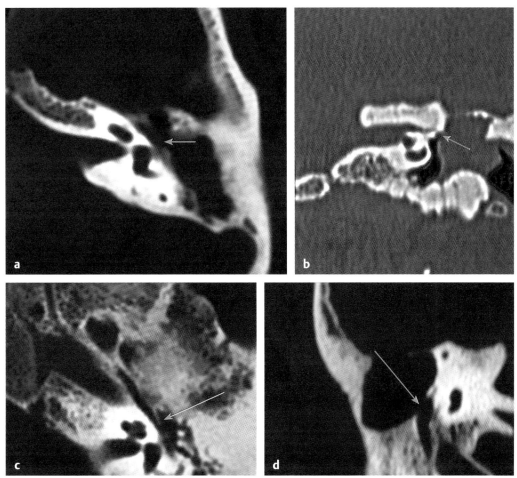

Fig. 16.7 High-resolution computed tomography (HRCT)—axial **(a)** and coronal **(b)** scans. In a patient with facial nerve palsy, *arrow* shows erosion of tympanic segment of facial canal (*arrow*). **(c)** In another patient, focal erosion of facial canal is seen (*arrow*). **(d)** In surgically proven case of cholesteatoma, erosion of facial canal near second genu (*arrow*) is noted.

Section D

Surgical Outcomes

17 Postsurgical Evaluation and Complications

This chapter illustrates different postoperative images. It is very important to audit one's own surgical results and to have proper documentation. The author recorded tympanic membrane after tympanoplasty, ossiculoplasty, and mastoid exploration. This will help to know the results of ossiculoplasty, fate of prosthesis, conditions of mastoid cavity, and different complications of otological surgeries.

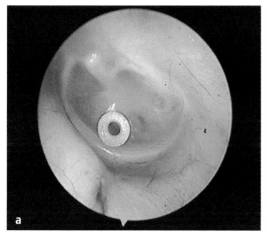 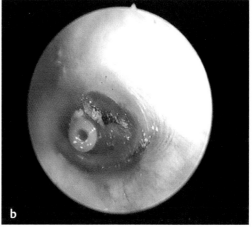

Fig. 17.1 **(a, b)** Shephard's Grommet is placed in anteroinferior quadrant of tympanic membrane. It was done for otitis media with effusion.

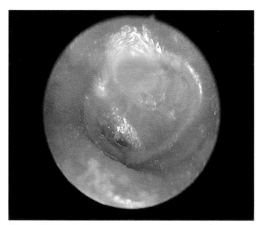 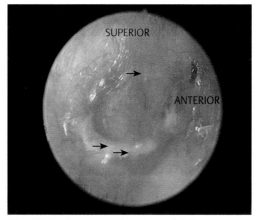

Fig. 17.2 Left ear tympanic membrane 4 months following tympanoplasty surgery. Note the fibrous annulus which is placed exactly at the bony annulus.

Fig. 17.3 Postoperative view of right tympanic membrane after tympanoplasty. Note the thickened fibrous annulus inferiorly, and neovascularization around handle of malleus.

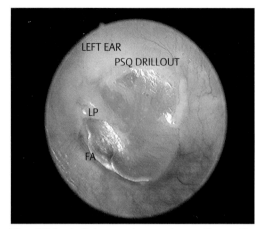

Fig. 17.4 Left tympanic membrane 6 months after tympanoplasty. Note the posterosuperior bony overhang drillout region. FA, fibrous annulus; LP, lateral process of malleus; PSQ, posterosuperior quadrant.

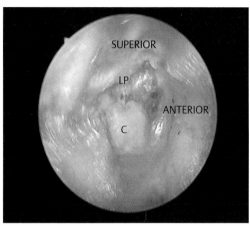

Fig. 17.5 Postoperative tympanic membrane of right side. This is a case of cartilage–island tympanoplasty. C, cartilage; LP, lateral process of malleus.

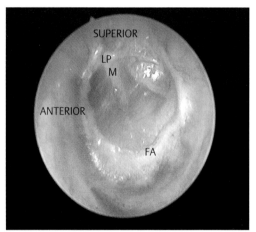

Fig. 17.6 Postoperative view of left tympanic Membrane. Note the beautiful orientation of fibrous annulus placed properly at bony annulus. FA, fibrous annulus; LP, lateral process of malleus; M, malleus.

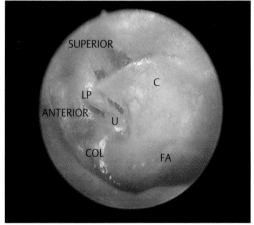

Fig. 17.7 Postoperative view of cartilage tympanoplasty done in a case of atelectatic otitis media. Thin sliced cartilage is placed posterior to malleus. One can notice adequate middle ear space after surgery. C, cartilage; COL, cone of light; FA, fibrous annulus; LP, lateral process of malleus; U, umbo.

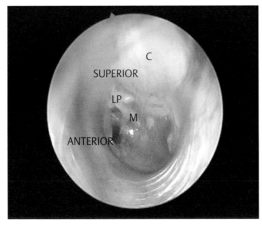

Fig. 17.8 Left tympanic membrane and cartilage reconstruction of attic. Thin slice of cartilage is placed at the region of posterosuperior drillout. C, cartilage; LP, lateral process; M, malleus.

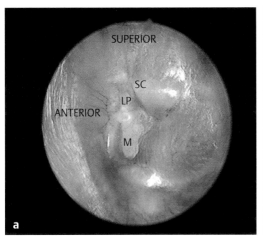

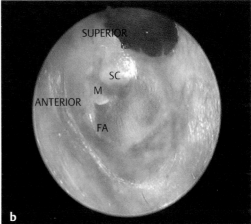

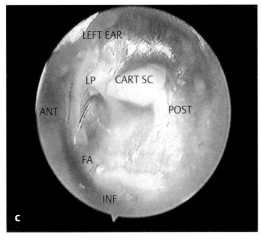

Fig. 17.9 **(a)** Postoperative view of ossiculoplasty of left ear. Sculptured auto incus short columella (SC) is seen through neotympanum. **(b)** Postoperative view of ossiculoplasty of left ear. Cartilage SC is seen through tympanic membrane. **(c)** Postoperative view of left ear ossiculoplasty. Cartilage short columella can be noticed through neotympanum. Note there is a space kept between a short columella and posterior annulus which is essential for good hearing. FA, fibrous annulus; LP, lateral process; M, malleus.

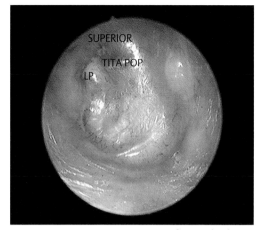

Fig. 17.10 Postoperative view of ossiculoplasty. Titanium partial ossicular prosthesis (TITA POP) is seen through the neotympanum. Cartilage cap is displaced and prosthesis is in direct contact with tympanic membrane. LP, lateral process.

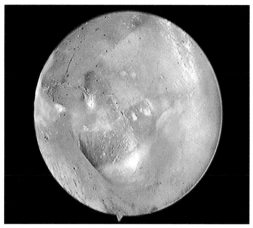

Fig. 17.11 Postoperative view of left tympanoplasty and attic reconstruction with sliced cartilage.

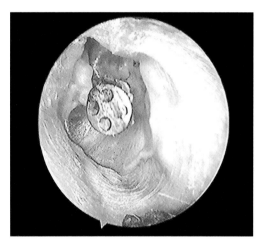

Fig. 17.12 Postoperative picture of titanium prosthesis extruding from neotympanum (left ear).

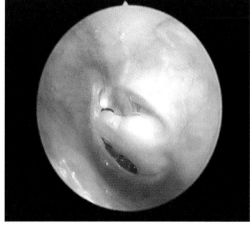

Fig. 17.13 Postoperative picture of left ear of cartilage tympanoplasty having a residual perforation at anteroinferior quadrant.

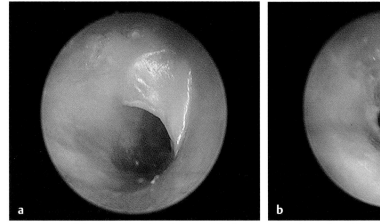

Fig. 17.14 **(a)** Postoperative photograph showing "L"-shaped cartilage extruding from middle ear. "L"-shaped cartilage is used when stapes suprastructure is absent. **(b)** Titanium prosthesis extruding through neotympanum keeping a residual perforation.

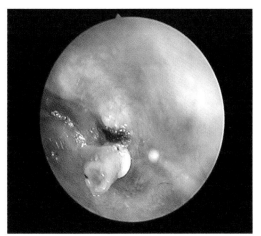

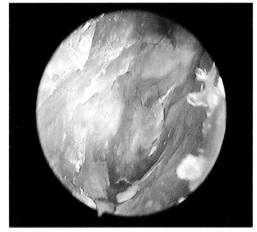

Fig. 17.15 Extruded polytetrafluoroethylene (PTFE) partial prosthesis in external auditory canal. This extrusion was a gradual process. One can notice the tympanic membrane was intact giving rise to type III tympanoplasty-like assembly. This patient had 20-dB air conduction threshold with less than 10-dB air-bone gap.

Fig. 17.16 Postoperative picture of right ear mastoidectomy with mastoid cavity obliteration with temporalis muscle pedicled flap. Note that it looks like a normal external auditory canal.

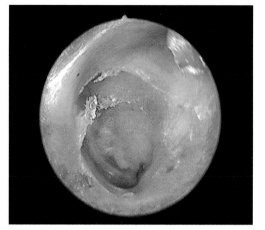

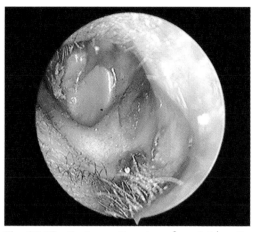

Fig. 17.17 This is a 4-month postoperative picture of mastoidectomy case. Musculo perio-steal flap obliteration of mastoid cavity gives smooth, healed, external auditory canal with almost no cavity.

Fig. 17.18 Postoperative view of mastoid cavity seen through adequate meatoplasty.

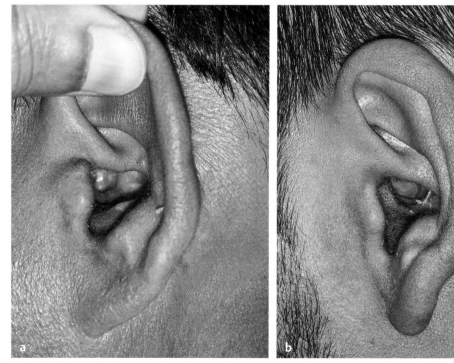

Fig. 17.19 (a, b) Photographs of "Just adequate meatoplasty." Meatoplasty should be done after cavity reconstruction and depending upon neocavity size.

Index